T0117140

The British Aestheticians Guide To

Waxing The Lady Garden

Claire Barnes

authorHOUSE®

AuthorHouse™
1663 Liberty Drive
Bloomington, IN 47403
www.authorhouse.com
Phone: 1-800-839-8640

Published by AuthorHouse 3/29/2012

ISBN: 978-1-4685-6159-3 (sc)
ISBN: 978-1-4685-6158-6 (e)

Library of Congress Control Number: 2012904672

This book is printed on acid-free paper.

Because of the dynamic nature of the Internet, any web addresses or links contained in this book may have changed since publication and may no longer be valid. The views expressed in this work are solely those of the author and do not necessarily reflect the views of the publisher, and the publisher hereby disclaims any responsibility for them.

Cover design by Carolyn Sheltraw, www.csheltraw.com.
Model in cover image is the author herself.

Preface

This is a follow on book from my first waxing book "The British Aestheticians Guide to Waxing the Twigs and Berries". Some of you may have been 'heck no' I have no desire to wax a guy's nether regions so maybe decided to never read it. Hence my reasoning for making a second edition for those not willing to delve into the man's junk yard department with your waxing stick!

To all my lovely professional readers who are licensed, or about to be licensed in the aesthetics trade, this isn't intended as your *only* training tool but one that should supplement DVDs and hands-on training classes with professionals already in the know before you let yourself loose on a paying client. Round up your friends and your existing clients, give out free waxing sessions, maybe even become 'legs up Lucy' and practice on yourself behind a locked door!

Actually being legs up Lucy is not as easy as you might think. I must admit I do have it down to a fine art though, it just takes forever. The best way to do it is by standing up and placing one foot on the bathroom counter in a sort of lunge position whilst standing on an old towel, so you don't drip wax all over the floor.....and the rest is up to you to explore your own hairy crevices with the wax!

Maybe all those years of me being a gymnast has enabled me to do it myself.

The content of this manual is meant to be informative in a fun and cheeky way and is focused primarily on how to wax the lovely Lady Garden, how to utilize your salon social skills, sales and etiquette. After attending different waxing classes and talking with lots of other professionals so that I could learn what to do and what *not* to do and watching DVDs, coupled with hands-on waxing of male and female body parts over the years, I learnt very quickly what worked best for *me*. So, please by all means, take this knowledge of wax and its wonderful capabilities with you to *all areas* of the female body throughout your waxing profession.

Make sure you have your technique up to high expectations before you charge your clients. Along the way, this guide is here to provide some tid-bits of valuable information that you maybe didn't pick up in beauty school or in other areas of training once you became licensed.

You may find that I repeat myself in the book. When I do this, I am doing it to keep reinforcing important things that you need to have memorized.

Also, please check that the state that you are licensed in is in acceptance of the services that you offer in your salon. All states within the U.S.A have their own rules and regulations when it comes to waxing.

Contents

Acknowledgements

I would like to give a big thanks to Carolyn Sheltraw my book illustrator and the man in Home Depot who was very patient with me, whilst I tried different hedge trimmers for size for the photo shoot for my front cover. Incidentally, the hedge trimmer that I bought I did return after the photo shoot as my condo balcony has no need for it….so I do apologize Mr Home Depot man if you lost your commission on 'said' item!

Big thanks to my boyfriend Drew Ferraro, who rolled his eyes at me when I announced I was working on book number two! Your patience is marvellous.

Very big thanks to both my children Dylan and Penny. I know being teenagers you are oblivious to what is going on around you, unless it involves you, but thanks for your patience whilst I wrote the book (if you didn't already notice or know that I was writing instead of attending only two soccer games that week and not the usual four!) Love you both dearly, warts and all!

Thanks for the support that I got from previous readers of my first book "The British Aestheticians Guide to Waxing the Twigs and Berries". Your encouragement and compliments pushed me to producing this book.

Also, thank you to all people involved in "The Real Life" section of the book. Sharing your stories probably took up a good part of your day. For this I hug you! Hugs also for those who endorsed the book .... Jennifer Johnston (Waxbitch), Andy Rouillard from Axiom Bodyworks in the U.K and Crickett (The Wax chick)

Change is inevitable, growth is intentional.
Glenda Cloud

What is the
Lady Garden?

Quite simply, this is a cheeky, fun term that is often used in England to describe the private female body parts. In this manual, you may find that I use other typical British terminology to also describe things and you will find a glossary at the back of the book as a translation for you if I use any words that confuse you.

The Americans and the British may both speak English, but our terms and phrases we use can differ greatly.....

When waxing the Lady Garden it can consist of just the modest bikini area where the sides are just waxed or the whole nine yards down under -- as in a full Monty "Bob's your Uncle" and it's all gone sort of wax! So grab yourself a mirror and examine yourself down there to where you have hair as any of that can be removed skillfully and quickly by a confident aesthetician. Hopefully *you* will be that aesthetician!

What Can She Expect When Getting Her Waxing Service?

Your client should expect *some* discomfort, especially if it is her first time being waxed, and especially if it is her first time having her Lady Garden mowed. She should expect to work for her service by holding herself at times to allow you to apply the wax and remove it. She will need to stretch her skin to assist you in the process and bend her legs from time to time so that you can get into those nooks and safely remove the wax without hurting her or bruising the area. This is especially important if she is larger set.

Most clients tell me that the most painful part to be waxed is the top part around the pubic bone where the hair is denser. The labia, doesn't hurt as much as their pubic bone area does, especially if you pull the skin tightly. Pulling the skin taut is especially important if they have quite a loose labia area.

She will love the results and, once you get her hooked, there will be no going back. She may feel a bit tender for a few hours after she has had her waxing and even a bit of itching is to be expected. Send her home with a good soothing cream that your salon retails.

It has been noted from both male and females that when they are fully waxed down below, their sexual sensation greatly increases. This is a good *selling point* for you to use, especially if you have a client that is questioning the reason behind the advantage of going for the full Brazilian as opposed to the basic bikini wax. If she is at a point in her life, where her sex life might need some spice, you may have made a sale. Cha-ching!

Some clients wax this area because they like the clean feel to it, making them feel more hygienic. Some clients do it for sexual reasons. We as aestheticians are not there to question the reasons why they do it. We just do it!

It might also be a good idea to let your client know that once she has had a full wax down there going to the loo might seem a bit strange and might leave her wondering why her pee-pee 'stream' is not aiming into the toilet bowl, but seems to be showering herself instead! Hair down there helps control how the urine flows. Once the hair has been removed the stream loses its control slightly and *can* spray like a sprinkler system! So tell her to watch how she squats to avoid wet bum cheeks.

The Questionnaire

First, you will need to ask her to fill out a questionnaire. (Boring I know as most people hate it when they are handed those pesky things to fill in, and some of the questions seem to be completely irrelevant to the service or visit that they are participating in.) You know the ones with endless questions regarding what medications they are on, etc.

Acutane and Retin-A: If the client is using any of these lotions/medications for acne or fine lines, you will need to tell her to hold off on waxing for two weeks since she last applied the Retin-A and at least six months since she last used Acutane.

These products cause thinning of the skin as they are both Keratolytics. Keratolytics increase the speed of skin exfoliation and, even though they may use this product on the face for acne or fine lines -- and not necessarily around "The Lady Garden" -- the product 'migrates' which means it gets into the blood stream through the pores and just causes a whole array of problems when combined with waxing. Typically, when clients use these products and have a wax, the skin due to its sensitivity will burn. Sometimes the scars from the wax burn can also be permanent.

You will also have to ask her if she suffers from herpes or any other sexually transmitted disease (STD). This isn't because you are nosey; you just want to protect yourself and, more importantly, if your client is susceptible to these diseases, you don't want to spread it or bring on those little herpes buggers that might be lying dormant!

Your questionnaire should also consist of questions about whether they are on blood thinners, whether they are vitamin deficient, or if they take aspirin daily as aspirin is also a blood thinner. Knowing the answers to these questions helps you to be more aware of their potential to bruising.

Another question I think is important to ask is if they have a pacemaker, pregnant or if they are epileptic. I go into why I ask this question in Tip 10 on high frequency later in the book.

Some of the questions might seem pointless, but it is very important that we know the answers before any waxing service. From waxing eyebrows to the hairs on their toes, we need to understand what medications they are taking before we go ahead.

When she has filled out the form, be sure to then read it. Don't just take it for granted that she is Mrs. Clean Bill of Health. With any answers that she gives to you, spend some time with her and discuss any concerns or further questions that you may have.

You also need to inform your clients why you are asking these questions. There is nothing wrong with telling a client that using Retin-A when waxing can cause them to lose half their skin due to an increase in exfoliation that occurs, when using that medication. Unless the client is a real sassy miss, then they should understand why it is important to be honest – otherwise, they will pay the consequences.

We all have our little secrets, and, over the years, I have found that *it is* more likely to be a female client that tells little fibs about her use of Retin-A. Maybe they want people to think their flawless complexion and wrinkle-free face is all down to natural perfection, so they withhold from sharing this information. It is all good, but once you have explained to the client the reasoning behind your questions, we would hope that they would then fess up!

The number 'one' reason why salons or spa's are sued in the U.S.A is from 'waxing'! Protect yourselves and do not be complacent with your client's safety. It might come back to bite you!

Please read the chapter on all contraindications for waxing in general as it is important that you know these things and have these questions on your questionnaire form.

When is it too young to get a bikini wax?

Obviously the client has to be old enough to have reached puberty! No crazy parents dragging their daughters in to remove one or two hairs! It might sound crazy, but it has actually happened on a few occasions, both cases reaching the media due to its absurdity. The girl in question in one of the incidents was an eight year old, whose mother dragged her in for beautification down below. So the answer to this question is going to differ from person to person and eventually it will start to differ according to new laws and regulations depending on what state you live in, in the U.S.A.

California is the first state in America to make it illegal for a client to use a tanning bed if he/she is under eighteen. But there is no law as of yet as to what the minimum age requirement is for clients when receiving bikini waxing. This will change I am sure. I do know that most salons require clients to be sixteen years old before they can get a wax. This is more for insurance purposes than a legal issue. If they are under sixteen and something disastrous happened, your liability insurance for your salon probably wouldn't cover the costs.

So in my humble opinion I wouldn't do a full Brazilian bikini wax on a client under sixteen. This is to cover my own back from an insurance perspective, but also for the client herself. I personally feel in your salon you have to have a cut off point. Unfortunately there are some salons that do take them younger than that and that can be their cross to bear and I am glad I am not the one carrying it.

Girls are getting younger and younger now when it comes to having beauty treatments and the pressure is accelerating. I would be more comfortable knowing that I have set the boundaries and I am not having to deal with a crazy parent throwing a temper tantrum because I won't wax her thirteen year old.

As a parent of a fourteen year old daughter, it saddens me that girls younger than this are constantly looking for ways to improve their appearance to fit in with the crowd. Ok, if she had a huge bush growing out of the side of her bikini I would encourage her to trim it up a bit and get it groomed so it isn't unsightly. But, the whole removal of the Lady Garden at that age or younger is unnecessary, in my honest opinion.

When waxing the sixteen year old for her first time appointment I would insist that the client has a patch test done. I would apply some wax in one small area down below and remove it with my strip and send them home. Having a small area break out is better than having the whole Garden blossom into a blotchy mess. Within twenty four hours if there is no reaction, then go ahead and wax the rest of the area.

The age restriction policy for your salon should be in print on your menu and on the consultation form. It also prevents the receptionist from having to deal with any confusion at the front desk. Let them skip down the street to another salon, it's much better than having an irate father coming in demanding to know why you practically deflowered his thirteen year old daughter! Admittedly he might never find out, but if she was to develop a bad reaction, I am sure the beans would be spilt eventually. His princess wouldn't be the one getting the wrath, it would be *you*.

Contraindications
to All Waxing

Some doctors do not recommend waxing for people who are diabetic, have poor circulation or who have varicose veins. They are more likely to get an infection and should be advised to receive a doctor's note, prior to you waxing them.

Obviously, if they are just getting a bikini wax or brow wax, then they can be waxed if they have varicose veins. But, a leg wax is not advised especially if they have a lot of them. If they only have a couple, just avoid the area and certainly don't wax over them.

Pregnancy *can* be classed as a contraindication as during pregnancy there is a hormonal change and the skin can become more sensitive. I have heard of clients who got regular bikini waxes, then once pregnant had to stop this service as they broke out and became too sensitive to the wax. They were able to resume waxing once they were no longer pregnant and once the hormones had settled down. I have waxed many clients throughout their pregnancies until the day before they gave birth and I never came across this kind of sensitive reaction, but it can happen, so clients do need to be aware of this.

Wax should not be applied over these areas:

- Raised moles and skin tags
- Any abrasions, bruises, bites, stitches, or broken skin
- Psoriasis, eczema (especially inflamed areas)
- Acne with infected pustules
- Any scars from surgery which are less than six months old (hysterectomy, caesarean scars or an episiotomy from recent childbirth)
- Vasectomy scar less than six months old (if you are waxing the Twigs and Berries)

I once had a male client come in for a back wax. When I walked into the room and saw him lying face down waiting for me, I noticed his back was covered in long scratches on either side. I asked him if he had been wrestling a lion and what the heck had he done to his back! He informed me that he had a wild date the night before and she got a bit crazy during a night of passion!

I told him I wasn't really comfortable applying wax onto his back as some areas were slightly inflamed. He kept insisting that I waxed his back as he was going for round two that evening with the same girl and wanted to be 'groomed'. I am sure he probably went to another salon down the street because I said 'No'. I lost the service and the client, but I was happier this way as it was a risk I wasn't willing to take.

Just like you would never give a client a facial with a cold sore, I would also never encourage you to do a *lip wax* on a client if she has one. It will certainly irritate the cold sore and is a sure guarantee that it will make it spread. It has been said to never wax a client if they are even susceptible to cold sores, regardless of whether they have an outbreak or not as it can actually trigger one. I am blessed once a year with the curse of cold sores and I receive waxes all the time and have never found this to be the case. From a holistic standpoint cold sores typically start from the base of the spine! Yes, they start from the nerve endings at the base of the spine; usually due to stress, being over tired which causes a low immune system or from too much sun without SPF lip protection.

If you prefer in your salon to not offer waxing services to people who are *susceptible* to cold sores that is your call. Personally, if their outbreaks are once a year or once every couple of years, I would say it is pretty safe to go ahead with waxing. If they suffer from cold sores at least five times a year or more, it's probably best that they don't get this service.

I also once had another male client who came in for a back wax with a severe acne breakout. I consulted with him that applying wax would certainly irritate the skin, making his acne worse. I recommended that he received several back facials with me to help with the acne and then we could take it from there. I gained a new client and helped him with his acne which was a reward within itself. He soon became a waxing client once we had his acne under control. Knowing that he was a client with acne prone skin, we always used a cream wax specifically for sensitive skin.

Also, as mentioned earlier, if a client has a current genital herpes outbreak, then avoid waxing the labia area. Just out of courtesy, I would hope a client with a genital herpes outbreak, wouldn't *even* consider putting themselves or somebody else other than a doctor through that exposure anyway!

If a client is using Retin-A, Acutane, or any other medical grade topical cream for Acne, waxing is not recommended.

If your client is epileptic, pregnant has a pacemaker or metal implants just refrain from using high frequency following any waxing. I go into why this is crucial in the high frequency chapter.

Lip or brow waxing following a facial isn't a contraindication, but it's advisable to wax *before* a facial. The skin is super soft and beautifully hydrated after a facial and has more chance of lifting or being more sensitive due to the usage of steam, extractions, or exfoliation that it might have received.

When pesky Aunt Flow visits us ladies once a month it is not a contraindication to waxing but it does make us more sensitive, both mentally and physically and it is worth you knowing this as some clients who are super hypersensitive choose to wait a few days before or after their period before receiving a wax. We can be crabby enough as it is during this time and really don't need the added pain thrown into the mix!

As described in the previous chapter, age should be a contraindication and should be made clear on the consultation form like all the other contraindications described.

Nervous Client

If you have a nervous client, the best thing you can do is to talk to her. Ask her to describe her main concerns. Really listen to what she has to say, making eye contact to give her that reassurance that you are a caring aesthetician. If you show enough confidence, then she will very quickly confide in you. However, if a dithering aesthetician was fumbling around your bits, sweating profusely, and shaking her head in confusion due to total lack of confidence, wouldn't it make you want to grab your knickers and run right out of the room? I would!

As a professional technician, you must talk to your client confidently to help relieve any nerves that she may have. We are not checking out her Garden to see if she looks any different to us and taking notes. We are just observing what we see so we can determine hair texture, skin, warts, moles, fresh episiotomy scars or anything else that we see that we have to be prepared for ahead of time.

Your client is coming in to see you for an intimate close-up service so her bits and bobs will be exposed to you whilst you are performing the service. Some people like to cover the client up and work around a towel or disposable underwear to help keep their dignity somewhat in tact. Personally, I think all that fuss and stuff gets in the way of us trying to do our job. After all, your client has come in to have her pubic hair removed, so we need to do our job without stuff getting in the way of the nooks and crevices.

It's like going in for a haircut with a hat on and expecting your stylist to cut your hair around it. We are professionals and we are not there to stare at someone's anatomy and compare it to any other female client we saw previously that day or compare her to ourselves. If she only wants the sides of her bikini waxed and not the whole nine yards, then, by all means, keep the disposable knickers on, or she can just keep her own knickers on. Unless her knicker drawer contains nothing but Prada or Versace undies, then I would most certainly use the disposable ones!

We go through enough Pap Smears and pretty much get used to our Genealogical visits (even though we don't squeal with excitement when we have *that* appointment!) so for the most part our female clients are not too embarrassed. Our male clients getting this service might be shy at first when exposing their tackle, but they soon settle down when you build up confidence with them also.

We should always show a certain amount of etiquette in the salon. If your client doesn't feel that she is getting that, then she, as a customer, is within her rights to express and voice her concerns and change salons or technicians. It is very important to really try to get the client to relax. The more relaxed she is, the more relaxed her muscles will be, which makes everybody happy and in the right frame of mind to do it again! So please, be confident in your approach. Do your best as a professional to get her comfortable. Compliment her on her lipstick or her eye-shadow. Ask her if she works out (if she is slim of course…please, don't ask her that if it is quite obvious she has never stepped foot in a gym!) We all like to be rewarded verbally for our hard work, so if it looks like she is in good shape from working out then tell her so.

There are millions of Aestheticians out there, but it's the person, not the title as to why clients return.

Before the Procedure

Coffee, tea or any other stimulant help us occasionally wake up in the morning or help us unwind after a long day, but consuming too much of any stimulant before a waxing appointment will only lead to more squirming, squealing, and discomfort. Why?

It's because our bodies become more acidic, and they certainly become more sensitive with an increase in blood flow, which, in turn, can make that labia turn more red than necessary.

It is also a good idea to inform the client before her appointment that she can dull the nerve endings before the service by taking an aspirin or ibuprofen twenty minutes prior to the appointment. It really does help to do this, and I would highly recommend telling all of your clients this and especially if like I mentioned earlier Aunt Flow is paying her a visit that day! People's pain threshold is much lower in the morning than it is in the late afternoon. If she finds waxing totally unbearable, suggest that she comes in later in the day next time to see if that makes a difference.

Also tell her to use a body scrub twice a week prior to waxing and to scrub around the pubic area to help 'exfoliate' those dead skin cells away from around the hair follicle. This helps ease the hairs exit, this also helps prevent ingrown hairs - especially if she continues to use it following the waxing procedure. If she doesn't have a body scrub at home, then this is a perfect time to show her your retail department and advise her on the best sugar scrub that she can buy. Retailing those scratchy exfoliation mitts in bright colors are a great take home product for your clients to use also. They easily pop into the washing machine and can be used as an alternative to body scrubs. Give your clients some options.

Personally, I prefer that clients use a sugar scrub as opposed to a salt scrub (*unless they are using Epsom salts, which I cover in the how to remove ingrown hairs section of the book*) Sugar is kinder on the skin and less dehydrating than salt. Also, rubbing salt into skin, especially around that area, is asking for trouble. Tell her to wait for twenty four hours after her wax since rubbing sugar scrub into a freshly waxed area will be like rubbing your face up and down a hard bristle brush for five minutes. Exfoliating really does keep the follicle clean of dead skin, which then helps to discourage the hair from becoming ingrown.

I would advise against using a loofah due to their porous nature as they can harbour bacteria in the crevices. It is also surprisingly a good breeding ground for yeast to grow! They are also a bit too coarse for use in this area and should just generally be avoided.

It makes for a much better service if she hasn't shaved for at least two to three weeks so that the hair is long enough for the wax to grab onto. The hair ideally should be at least

¼ inches long. If the pubic hair is way too long and she looks like she is sporting a rain forest down there, then you might have to use clippers on it so it is easier to wax and less painful for her.

Some technicians do charge extra for using the clippers as it takes more time to complete the service. I prefer not to charge them as I feel it is all part of the preparation. You set the prices in your salon, so it is your call as to whether there is an add-on fee or not for clipping the hair down. But, I do think it is a good idea to have a variety of prices on our menu when waxing our clients. We don't charge per square foot, per se, but we should charge much more if she has never trimmed or waxed down there before. It will take you much longer to work through the jungle and this should be reflected in your pricing.

Another good reason for your client to not have super long hair down there is that when it is too long it might break at the surface of the skin (which is no different to shaving) and can break off during waxing. That hair needs to come out at the root.

Sometimes, when there are nice juicy roots with a big bulbous end, it can be pretty cool to show your client the waxing strip so that she can see that waxing is all worthwhile and when done properly, it does work! Most clients don't like to see their own hair stuck to a muslin strip, but some do ask.

Ok, I know that skinny jeans have made a come back, and on some of our clients, they look great, but try and get her to leave those at home and opt for the loose, cotton trousers or skirt from her wardrobe instead. Chaffing isn't good after waxing and plucking at your jeans trying to loosen them out of a chaffed crack isn't particularly feminine and can make her very sore!

Wearing tight jeans following a Lady Garden wax can make her more prone to getting a yeast infection. The hair is there for a reason but due to cosmetic reasons we still ignore this fact as getting waxed down there does make you feel cleaner and sexier. From time to time it is our prerogative to ignore these medical facts, but be warned as vanity can come with a price!

So, advise your clients to arrive, clean and loose, and ready to breathe (physically and mentally). It is nice that they may want to smell all nice and sweet before they disrobe, but, hopefully, she will stay clear of lotions as too much lotion can make it oily down under and we will prep the skin the professional way, not her way.

Consulting with the first time waxing client about hair length, comfortable clothing, and caffeine intake is always better when the receptionist makes the confirmation call or when initially booking the appointment. This isn't because the fashion police are prowling the salon or because we have more rules than we know what to do with. Instead, this is for the client's comfort, which should be our priority. It's just much better for her to know these simple instructions prior to coming into the salon, especially if she is a virgin to waxing so that she can then plan ahead of time.

I used to have a regular client who came in monthly for her

wax with a skirt on. After her wax she kept her knickers in her handbag and she used to share with me at her next visit how excited her husband was to learn that she was driving home with her skirt on all knickerless and sexy! The things clients share with you, hey?

Enthusiasm is contagious. Be a carrier.
Susan Rabin

Table Set-up

Here is what you need to have on-hand for your waxing service:

- Double wax heater or, if your room is large enough to hold a four-wax heater, all, the better…..
- Hard waxes
- Soft waxes
- Strips
- Hundreds of spatulas (as I don't recommend double dipping …nasty)
- Powder
- Prep oil
- Magnifying lamp
- Numbing spray (if you choose to use it prior to the waxing)
- Numbing lotion (if you choose to use it following the waxing)
- Disposable cleansing cloths
- Cleansing lotion
- Soothing lotion
- Latex gloves
- Sanitary wipes
- Tweezers (good aestheticians shouldn't rely on these…she's in for a wax, not a tweezing!)

- Jar of Barbicide® (for sanitizing tweezers/clipper blades)
- Clippers (if she is sporting a 70's bush)
- Towels
- High frequency machine
- Facial gauze (if using high frequency)
- Massage heat pad (optional)
- Vajazzling jewels (if you are adding this to the service)

So, now that we have the table set up, the room is of a comfortable temperature for both of you -- not too hot, not too cold. This is for your comfort and also hers, but it is also crucial to the temperature and application of the wax.

If she is too hot, she will sweat and trying to apply wax onto sweaty skin can make you sweat in frustration, which leads to a big sweaty situation and the room will resemble a skinned cat fight in a sauna.

If the room is too cold, she will be shivering, you will have ice cold hands even through the gloves, and the wax temperature can make the wax get too thick, which will be a blobby, stiff, and big sticky mess. Situations like this do happen as things can go wrong – it's the nature of the beast!

Out of courtesy to your client, I think it is always nice to check in with them about how comfortable they are in regards to the room temperature. In some salons that I have worked at I have used a nice electric heat pad hidden under the sheets. Some clients like the soothing heat on their backs when they are having a facial or a wax. If the temperature in your room is usually quite warm and you don't have the option of adjusting it, then a heat pad is probably not a good idea as they will get too hot. Play it by ear as to how the client feels, reassuring her that at any time you can turn the heat down or off if need be. Those extra miles of customer service can make all the difference.

I also think it's nice to ask a client if they are happy with the music that you have playing. Most say "yes" and don't expect you to spin tunes like a top DJ and play requests for them, but it's nice for the client to be asked and it all makes for a top-notch customer service reputation for your salon or spa.

Admittedly, if it is not your own place of business but you are an employee with no choice as to what music is playing, then you are probably best keeping your mouth shut and not bringing attention to the situation *and* so you don't get into a pickle with your boss about his/her choice of music playing throughout the salon. But some employers allow you to have an iPod® docking station in your room where you can choose your own tunes, or better still if you rent the room, then, the music is all yours!

While we are on the subject of client comfort, please make it your duty to avoid phone calls during the service. She may not be having a relaxing facial with dolphins playing in the background, but she is still spending money and expecting a service from you. Answering your cell phone or texting during any service is rude and is a sure guarantee that your client will not return.

If your phone accidentally bellows out the National Anthem, apologize to your client and switch your phone off or put it on silent! If you suspect it could be an emergency (as these do happen) then politely dismiss yourself to answer the call out of the room. If it isn't a life or death situation, return to the room promptly with the phone off and again apologize to your client.

I once felt like the third person during a hair cut that I had with a girl who took it upon herself to answer a personal phone call during my service. I was there for a service; I was short on time and felt that she was totally dismissive of my time while she chatted for a few minutes. It is not necessary and makes your client feel very unwanted. She began to proceed cutting my hair with "Ooh, where was I?" No apology, nothing! If you don't have a receptionist to make your appointments for you, allow your voicemail to take all messages and return them when you are in between clients.

Meeting Her at Reception/ Salon Etiquette

Always greet your client with a nice smile and a relaxed confident, happy manner.

If it is the first time that you are meeting her, you only have a few seconds to form a lasting impression so make sure you "wow" her with your pizzazz. The general public forms an opinion based on someone's looks within seven to twenty seconds. Even if it is your third time meeting the client, you should still treat her like she is your *only* client.

Become an actor in your environment and set the performance for each client that walks onto your stage. The most successful service technicians are ones that do this. They recognize that their personal problems have to be left at home and the stage has to be set and ready for action each time an existing or new client comes to you for a service. I admit this can be tiring and sometimes by the end of the day our faces are so transfixed into this permanent wedged Wallace and Gromit smile where our jaw line feels like it will never fall back into place again easily, but as part of our profession we always have to keep on smiling.

The general public judges others based on looks, body language and attitude more than anything else. You have one chance to create a long lasting impression, so the rule as always is dress for success. Your appearance reflects how you feel about yourself, so you should be clean and very professional and your hair tied off your face if you have long hair. There should not be a trace of spinach in your teeth as, hopefully, you will have freshened up, and your smile should dazzle her to show her your true brilliance!

While we are on the subject of teeth, if you are a smoker it is strongly advisable to visit your dentist regularly. There is nothing worse than coming face to face with a person and their breath smells like they have had camel dung sandwich for lunch. So regardless of whether you smoke, or indulge in lots of garlic, keep a spare toothbrush at work with you to avoid any embarrassing halitosis moments!

An old beauty school teacher of mine once told us in class that most clients who visit salons or spas are spending at *least* $50 each visit, so, at the very least, you should look like you have spent at least that amount on yourself. Competition is very close to home. Winning your clients over within the first twenty seconds is crucial. We don't always get a second chance.

I have always found in the past that when I was wearing a nice, classy uniform for work, or an eye-catching 'sassy' apron, that during my down time from clients, I would get asked where did I work? What did I do there? So, in your down time in between appointments, head to the grocery store to pick up your lunch or pop into your nearby coffee place and let people start the conversation with you. This will then give you the opportunity to hand out your business cards and network. This is a really good idea for the 'shy' aesthetician, who isn't great at marketing herself. Sell yourself by the way that you dress and have *them* approach you. You never know, you might get a date out of it too!

If your client enters the salon and you roll your eyes because the magazine that you were reading was at a juicy point and then you reluctantly throw your magazine down and, like a limp fish, shake her hand (if she is *even* lucky enough to get a handshake) and then mumble under your breath the introduction, you will have created an impression. The impression would have been "You are not that into your job, you don't care about her, and your magazine is way more interesting than what she is." Good job, sister!! ☹

You must look at every client that walks through your door as your ideal client and treat them as such. Never make them feel that they are an interruption to your day or a big fat inconvenience. People who walk through your door are a word-of-mouth machine that can spread the word about your location, good or bad. At every point of engagement with your clients, you are essentially marketing your business.

You could do the best, most efficient service on her when she is in the treatment room, but her first impressions are what she encountered and are what she will remember. If your "meet and greet" skills are fantastic and your skill level is also fantastic in the waxing room, you are sure to get a repeat client and, better still, a client who recommends your services to her friends. Cha-ching!

So, be genuine and warm at all times. When you consider what each client means to your future and your bank account, then this shouldn't be so difficult. Practice these skills often enough and it will very soon become second nature.

I learnt a very important lesson from somebody a while back who told me that "your brand is not your logo, it is not your company name, it is not necessarily what you wear (even though these all do contribute and play an important role), BUT it is how you made them feel!" This is who people buy from and this is what people remember when they think of you. Author Dale Carnegie once said "We are evaluated and classified by four contacts: what we do, how we look, what we say, and how we say it".

So, greet your client, shake her hand or just place a gentle hand on her arm, and introduce yourself, making eye contact with her. Give her the reassurance she needs just by you being confident. Don't underestimate the power of using her name even if it is a difficult one to pronounce. Focus for a few seconds on the name or form a picture in your head to form an association with it so that you don't make the mistake of forgetting it. Some people understandably get upset if you keep forgetting their name.

During the service, use her name a couple of times to secure that you as a technician can bond with the client. Whenever I discuss etiquette in this book, I want you to always put yourself in your client's shoes and think of different scenarios that *you* may have encountered. Were you made to feel neglected or unimportant? Or were you made to feel appreciated or overwhelmed by fantastic customer service? You decide which role you want to play in regards to how much salon etiquette you possess. Your client's safety and happiness followed by your retention rate, your bank account, and your tip jar is what should be important to you and all in that order.

It is reasonable to assume that if your tone of voice is happy, or excited, you will be able to project a more favourable impression than if your tone of voice is bored, frustrated, resentful or just tired. So, take the gum out of your pie hole, speak clearly and hopefully with teeth free of spinach, you will have given her a good first impression. I could waffle on all day about spa/salon etiquette and how important it is today as I know what works and what doesn't.

I have worked in low-end salons to very high-end hotels and the rule applies everywhere. People do business with people they like and trust. Some of you reading this may be thinking, "What? Does she think I am an idiot? Of course I greet the client this way." But, surprisingly enough, not everybody does know or do this!! And, more importantly, some do it but not on a *consistent* basis.

I have been around the block often enough to come across the ones who "just don't get it!" So, my hopes are with writing this book, that those who just *don't get it* read this and think "maybe today is the day that I should get it, as the economy is tight, business might be going down the drain, and I need to step up to the plate and brush up on my people skills!"

Some technicians (and I have had technicians who have done it to me) become complacent and become too familiar, treating me like I am their friend. You are not their friend as such; they are your client. At anytime, a client can decide, for whatever reason, that they want to go somewhere else. It could be due to financial issues, personal issues, or that they just merely want a change. Either way, it affects your back pocket and can become personal when it doesn't need to be. So, keep treating them at each visit, like it is their first visit.

Female technicians with other female clients especially form this bond. When we have seen a client many times we start to share information, we share our feelings and our thoughts on a somewhat intimate level. Once we have formed this relationship with them we have similar thoughts with them as we do with men once we have had sex with them. We automatically presume "relationship, or love, or commitment" Once we form this bond with our clients, it can become more personal than it ever needs too when that client doesn't come to see us anymore. As I state above they can decide at any time that they do not wish to come to see you anymore. Make your work life easier by absolutely forming relationships with these clients, but compartmentalize in your brain where they fit into your *friendship* circles. Anytime you rely on somebody by way of an exchange of money, it is a different form of friendship. Keep it this way to avoid any unnecessary hurt, so you don't take it personally.

To me a friend is a friend who will pick you up from the airport when you are stranded at 2a.m, she will be the person who cooks me spaghetti and brings it over to my house when I am sick with snot hanging out of my nose. Do you expect this from your clients?

Joe Gonzales who wrote "The Hairdresser's Guide to Success" states in his book that:

68% of clients leave because they feel an *attitude of unconcern or indifference* on the part of the company and its employees.
15% leave because they are dissatisfied with a service or product
9% leave for competitive reasons
5% form other relationships
2% move away
1% die.

One recent study in his book also showed that 96% of customers never complain when dissatisfied, but 91% never come back. Another study showed that one unhappy client will tell an average of nine people about their dissatisfaction with a therapist and salon. Don't be that person or salon that has negative energy buzzing around the city about you as it can be devastating to your career's progress and financial growth.

I once overhead my hair stylist that I had been seeing for three years comment to the receptionist that she was really running behind. She started to say "Claire won't mind, she is super sweet"! Thanks for saying I am super sweet, but please, don't presume that you running late is *ok* with me. I didn't have plans for that afternoon, but I could have done. It made me feel that my appointment and the money that I paid for it, including the tip was just not appreciated. That day I didn't feel super sweet, I felt super sour! She was showing a perfect example of what Joe Gonzales relates to in the above statistics of *unconcern and indifference.*

Another big question you may have is "What do I address her by?" Do you call her "Mrs so and so?" Or do you address her by her first name. Your salon/spa will have its own branding and that should set the tone. Most high-end hotels require you to greet your clients in the spa by using "Miss" or "Mrs so and so." Only you and your salon will know the correct way to address your clients.

Everyone has a brand and it is called your reputation. It really does determine how people respond to you and whether they will listen to you, buy from you and return back to you.

Help her with her coat complimenting her on how nice it is or how great the color is on her. Be *sincere* in your approach and not too gushy as anybody will see through this. Ask her "what was the name of your lipstick again?" let her see you making a note of this. It shows you pay attention.

He who praises everybody insincerely, praises nobody!

She trusts you, as a professional, to have an aura of confidence about you. Shaking hands or a gentle touch on the arm whenever conducting business dictates you are forming a relationship with her. The service should end this way when she is at the reception area also so that you give the impression that you are grateful for her business with the hopes of seeing her again.

We are given two ears and one mouth for a reason....
use what we are given wisely.
Epictetus

Client Hygiene

Believe me, in our careers, we have or we will see or smell a Garden that is not as fresh as a daisy or sweet smelling like a freshly mowed lawn! So to avoid any embarrassment on both parts, please get her to wipe up properly with the wipes that you provide for her so that she can refresh her nether regions -- as it is not our job to remove any dingle berries! Most clients do freshen up before they arrive, but you will get the occasional client who is oblivious to her own hygiene.

There is nothing wrong with you putting on your consultation form a cute little reminder that *"All clients are much more appreciated if their Garden is sweet smelling like freshly mowed grass with good hygiene rather than a client who has an aroma like a heap of compost"*. Ok, maybe you don't need to be that blunt. But keep it fun so as to not be offensive and get the message across that way. It brings a pleasant reminder to the client that they need to do this before they expect you to stick your head down there and perform a waxing service on them.

I am sure they will get the hint if you applied a gas mask onto your face during the wax preparation process, but it will make it much less embarrassing for all involved if you just supply her with wipes. I couldn't even begin to tell you where you would even purchase a gas mask anyway, but we all know where we can buy wipes from.

When leaving the room, to give her a bit of privacy, you should provide her with a towel to cover up with, so that the Lady Garden is not exposed to the whole salon or to anybody just casually walking past the door! Our gynaecologist sees us naked from the waist down, but they don't stay in the room and watch us undress. They leave the room and provide a cover up to protect us from a lost patient accidentally walking into the room or passers by peeking in. So, to protect your client's nudity against strays walking in accidentally, leave the towel so she can cover up.

Client Consultation

Make sure she is in there for a Brazilian wax and not just an underarm wax! We all know from time to time that our very busy wonderful receptionists can make a mistake or things are just misunderstood over the phone. The last thing you need is to start prepping her downstairs department when she is wondering what the heck this has to do with her hairy armpits. She doesn't want any surprises!

Consult with her as to what her requirements are whilst she is in the room. Does she just require a very conservative bikini wax, where we only remove hair from the sides or does she want a landing strip left? Listen to what her requirements are and advise whenever possible if you have any other recommendations. Maybe, she might request a shamrock designed into her pubic hair for St Patricks Day or a heart if it is Valentines Day. Maybe, you wouldn't even know where to start with doing topiary designs on her lawn and she needs to know this beforehand. Not all aestheticians do have these stencils in stock or even know how to use them.

It is your job to find out this information and not to assume. *Whenever we ASSUME .... You basically make an ASS out of U and ME!*).

I will share a story with you that happened to me years ago when the Brazilian first became popular with females. I met my client in the reception area and she was booked in for a Brazilian wax. She was a rookie to the service and obviously when booking her appointment thought that the Brazilian was just a simple bikini wax.

During the procedure, I started to ferret my way through her Lady Garden, removing every inch of her pubic hair, whilst she was positioned in every yoga position known to man. She then started to panic and got slightly upset as she sat upright and, with a total look of sheer horror on her face, told me that she only wanted the sides done around her bikini area and then asked me why I insisted that she roll over so I could get her back passage!

I stood, rooted to the spot with the deer in headlights look on my face and with mouth gaping wide open like I was catching flies! I kept glancing down at the trash can, overflowing with spatulas and used wax strips with the hopes that somehow, *just somehow*, I could miraculously glue it all back on again and make it all right.

With my bottom lip quivering, I attempted to start explaining what I thought she was in for and that she should have been more clear during her time of booking the appointment, BUT I stopped myself before I made her feel like I was the victim. So, I just outright humbly apologized and told her how bad I felt that I didn't take the time to double check with her what exactly she was booked in for.

Some people have a hard time apologizing and are very

quick to point the blame at others. We cannot do this with our clients, we have to treat them like they are right…as difficult as it can be, it is detrimental to your business if you blame your clients and make them feel that they are in the wrong.

My consultation in the room didn't even take place, and I failed miserably! There was obviously no charge to the client. I didn't see her again and neither did I get a tip. *Actually, yes, I did get a tip. The tip is CONSULT with your client what their needs are!* Be clear before you start, so she isn't left resembling a plucked turkey for Thanksgiving as maybe she just wants to leave feeling like she still looks like an adult and not a new born baby.

Client Responsibility

Even though she may be paying top dollar for the service and may think she just has to lay there and think of England/America or whatever country she is from, she has to work with you so that she gets the best, quickest, and less painful encounter ever. By this I mean she is responsible for holding herself at times or holding her stomach up tightly or pushing down on her thigh to keep the skin taut. This is especially important if she is heavy set. I have had clients before where the skin was too loose around the legs and stomach area and it makes it much easier for both of you if there is assistance.

But, more importantly and I cannot say this enough, be confident and make her feel special. As in all walks of life, the more confident we are as individuals, the more confidence we instil in others. The more we make people feel special the more likely they are to return to us.

*The customer in every walk of business has to be made to feel like she is your **only** customer. If you accomplish this, you will be very successful. Even if your client has been a client for years, she should still be made to feel this way.*

Complacency breeds ignorance, which affects our bottom line.

If she has never had any *landscaping* before down there and her bush resembles something that you would find in the Amazon rainforest, it is strongly suggested that you get the clippers out or hedge trimmer, weed-wacker, or whatever you can get your paws on. Trim it down to a No. 2. As I mentioned earlier, if the hair is too long, it can break off at the skin's surface, so a nice ¼ inch is the ideal hair length.

So, once the consultation is out of the way and the possible trimming then it's time to get down to the nitty-gritty and begin prepping the skin for the application of wax.

Why We Wear Gloves

As we enter the room and our client is lying there with the towel over her, clean and wiped down from the baby wipes -- we then put on our latex gloves. We do not remove the towel, take a peek, and then put on the gloves. I strongly suggest putting your gloves on *before* you remove the towel.

Think about this -- if somebody was to remove the towel from your bits, take a peek, and then put on the latex, you would be thinking "hmmm, do I look like I have something going on down there that needs the latex?" So, before you engage in physical contact with your client, out of professionalism, please do this. You will actually be surprised as to how many technicians don't wear gloves during waxing as they find they get in the way, get sticky, and just annoy the heck out of them.

Again, think of the gynaecologist. They should have their gloves on before they remove our paper sheet, and they certainly don't go touching our downstairs Lady Garden without gloves on. Neither should you! Latex gloves protect us from diseases, blood spots, and Hepatitis C.

Latex gloves also protect the client. The nails, no matter how short they are, are a wonderful source of bacteria.

The most common bacteria found under the nail bed are 'staphylococcus.' It is nasty and can cause various skin diseases, including 'impetigo,' which is extremely contagious and spreads very quickly. Impetigo occurs when there is a break in the skin, but can also occur if there is no visible break in the skin. Bacteria enter the skin and grow there, causing inflammation and infection. Blisters occur and fill with pus; it is very unsightly and can be pretty painful.

When the hair is pulled from the root, it is very susceptible to infection. Wearing the latex gloves helps eliminate as much of this as possible. Blood spots can also occur with any type of waxing, which is a good enough reason in itself to wear gloves. If you do find your gloves get a bit sticky whilst waxing, sprinkle a bit of baby/corn powder over them, rub your hands together, and it will help with the tacky feeling. Hopefully, you won't be on such a tight budget that a fresh pair can't be replaced also.

Even though we are wearing gloves when we wax, it is also a good idea to double check that our immunizations are up to date. As aestheticians work so closely with the skin and sometimes use sharp implements like lancets* during facials (*depending on the State you are licensed in) it's advisable to have a Tetanus Shot, and a Hepatitis A and B shot. Unfortunately there is no shot available at the time of writing this book for Hepatitis C.

Hepatitis is a virus that is found in infected blood, semen, vaginal fluids and saliva. The disease causes liver damage, long term disease, liver cancer and death.

If an aesthetician waxed me wearing gloves, I would also consider going to see her for facials, if she did indeed offer this service. If she didn't wear gloves and tried to introduce me to a new facial service she was offering with a wonderful discount, I would most certainly refrain from taking her up on her offer. Who knows how many Lady Gardens, or Twigs and Berries she had touched that day. As aestheticians we all know to wash hands before and after every new client, but I don't want to take the risk, in case it just *slipped* her mind!

I've got a theory that if you give hundred percent all of the time, somehow things will work out in the end.
Larry Bird

Skin Prepping

Make sure your facial/massage bed is at a comfortable height for you to begin waxing. Ergonomics are something we should always take into account. If your bed is too low and you find that you are bending down constantly, it can affect your health over the long term. Ideally, flat shoes should be worn and not heels (I can be guilty of this occasionally as I just love heels), but, ideally, flat shoes arc better for the posture when waxing all day.

The lighting in the room should be sufficient enough also, so that it doesn't strain your eyes and the better the lighting the more hairs that you can see. Use your magnifying light during the waxing and also during the skin prepping time to check the area for hair growth patterns, or anything that might look dodgy!

Using a nice skin prep solution on your cleansing cloth, clean the area thoroughly to make sure the surface is clean and free from bacteria and also free from oil that the body naturally produces from its sebaceous glands.

Don't use a toner or astringent (certainly not alcohol!) as this will tighten up those little pores and squeeze the living daylights out of the hair follicle, which will make it harder to pull out the hair from its follicle. It also makes the skin too dry, which can cause lifting (another word for saying "pulling off the skin").

A nice warm towel over the area can be applied prior to the skin prep solution. This can help relax the client, but the warmth can actually help soften the pores, which helps ease the hair out of the follicle. So, killing two birds with one stone can only make your life and her life easier.

There are two ways to prep the skin prior to waxing: Prep oil or baby powder/corn starch. Some clients also like you to use a numbing spray or lotion before you start waxing them. If it is their first time -- and I can tell that they are nervous -- then I always use one before I wax. I tell the client that I am using it so that it helps to relieve some of the sting for them.

They do appreciate this extra kindness that you put into the service, and all the little extra things that you do will make her more likely to return to you and become more generous in the tipping department.

Of course, you are always going to come across a client who is as tight as a drum no matter what you do and moths fly out of their wallets when money has to be spent. Don't take it personally; as it is not always down to you, it is just the way that they are.

<u>Oil</u>

Ok, now some people like to use prep oil before waxing. Some of you may be asking, "prep oil before waxing? How can oil be applied to the skin before waxing?"

The reason we apply oil before waxing is to ensure that the skin is protected and only the hair is removed. After all, removing skin isn't what she is in for. If she was, she would be down at the plastic surgeon and having a skin lift or graft. We are here to wax and not remove the skin.

Also, some aestheticians like to use just powder before waxing and both are okay as it is all just a matter of preference.

Personally, I find that every client is different. I can usually tell this by their ethnic background. If they have what seems like oily skin, then I will apply powder as oily skin and prep oil is just a bad combination. If your client has dry skin and appears to have some flaky skin down there, then using powder will be too drying, so stick with using a small amount of oil. Skin that is dry is more prone to lifting, so prep your client accordingly. You will probably find that you steer towards one more than the other. If your client appears very nervous, she may be prone to sweating more, so avoid oil and use powder instead.

When applying oil to the skin prior to waxing, use a tiny amount. Put it in the palm of your hands, blot your hands against a clean towel to prevent too much application, and start dabbing the area down there with your palms to be waxed. If it feels too slick and shiny after you have applied it and she is starting to look shiny use a towel again, dab around the area to absorb any excess oil. The skin shouldn't feel oily at all. Neither should you see it glisten. In this case, less is better.

Powder/corn starch

Powder adheres to the hair and protects the skin. This is a perfect prepping method to use on areas that need to be waxed where the skin is thin, sensitive or sweaty. Powder is used on eyebrows, lips, and bikini areas to protect the skin from lifting.

When applying powder to the skin prior to waxing, use a light mist over the area so that you just coat the area lightly. If you use too much powder, the wax will form a sort of curdle-like consistency and it will just result in a poor application with bad hair removal. You can sprinkle the powder from the container over large body parts when waxing, but when waxing the facial area, always, always, apply powder to eyebrows or lips from powder sitting in your hand, never directly from the container itself!

Some wax companies advise you to not use powder with their wax as it is not needed. I still use the powder very sparingly before the application and have never encountered any problems. Check with the waxing company's educator on their protocol.

Tell your client what you are doing and why just out of courtesy and also as a confidence booster, especially if this is her first time. She will appreciate you telling her the reasons why you are applying powder and why you are doing what you are doing.

Clients don't make a point of doing business with technicians that they dislike, don't trust, or whom they have no respect for.

Applying the Wax

There are lots of different waxes to use. Wax comes in lots of different types, depending on hair textures/skin sensitivity, etc. If you are lucky enough to have a wax heater that holds several different pots of wax, then you can really play around with the different types of wax and enjoy seeing how they all work in relation to each client with different hair textures, etc.

Briefly discuss with your client the sort of wax you are using and why. Keep it to layman's terms and don't bore her with the chemistry of the wax (even if you know it). She just wants the simple facts without the fuss. Explaining to her which wax you are going to use and why will tell her that you are quite capable of doing your job and have it all under control. It also shows that you care about her and her well-being.

I personally like to start from the top and work my way down, using soft wax around the pubic area *leaving* a few inches in a circular shape around the pubic bone where I later apply the hard wax. She can pull her stomach up or push down on her thighs using firm pressure to allow you to apply wax and remove the wax whilst the skin is being kept taut. Keeping the skin taut makes application and removal so much easier.

This area and the bum cheeks (if she has a hairy bum) are the *only* part of the Brazilian wax where I use soft wax (with strips). I am not an advocate for soft wax in this area. If it works for you and you can do it efficiently and safely on your client without any harsh pulling, tugging or bruising then kudos to you!

So, instruct her in a friendly manner what her role is so that you can then begin to apply the application of the wax and begin her service.

Now, remember to use a clean spatula each time you dunk into the wax pot as double dipping can cause contamination. I say 'can' because I don't think it has ever been proven that double dipping has done this before.

To be on the safe side, I would stick with (excuse the pun) the State Board rules and regulations and get into the habit of using clean spatulas/sticks for each dip just to prevent cross contamination if nothing else. I do go into detail a bit later in the book about the importance of no double dipping.

I wouldn't like to think I was having a lip wax with wax that had earlier been in contact with a not so clean Lady Garden or a man's Scrotum.

Always test the temperature of the wax on your inside wrist before you begin. It should be as close to body temperature as possible. If it feels hot to the touch, then it is too hot to apply to the downstairs body parts or any part of the body for that matter. Turn the temperature down if it is too hot and leave it to cool slightly with the lid off. If the wax also literally drips off the spatula and is of a very runny consistency, that is a good guideline that the wax is too hot to apply to the body also.

The same rule applies to hard wax also. Hard wax at the right temperature is easy to roll around the spatula, leaving a bulbous blob at the end with no rapid dripping. If the hard wax in the tin is the same consistency and all runny, it is also too hot. Hard wax at the right temperature has a thicker centre with the outside less firm, but certainly not drippy!

When you have the soft wax at the perfect temperature, you can then begin waxing your client. Dip your clean disposable spatula into the wax. On the one side of the stick, wipe the excess off on the side of the waxing rim. Hopefully, you have a paper collar around the pot to catch any drips. A soiled, sticky pot is also a good breeding ground for bacteria and a State Board faux pas, so use a paper collar and change it frequently.

Apply firmly a thin layer of soft wax to the skin, holding the stick at a 90-degree angle, and with the other hand, stretch the skin ever so lightly as you do this so that the spatula doesn't drag and blob too much wax in one place onto the skin. As you hold the skin taut, the wax application is thinner and this makes hair removal so much better.

Holding the skin taut whilst applying wax and removing wax helps to prevent hickies, love bites, or what ever term you are familiar with. If you apply soft wax too thickly, this puts too much pressure on the skin and can also cause bruising when removing the strip. So keep your soft wax thin!

Hold the skin around the area that you are about to wax and pull taut whilst applying the wax *in the direction* of the hair growth. Apply wax in very small sections until you pick up your speed. If you apply wax to the hair in the opposite direction to the natural hair growth pattern, as you pull the strip off, it will break the hair at the surface, leaving dark spots (these are not blackheads, but broken hair).

Keep your sections small and continue checking on the direction of the hair growth when applying the wax. Personally, I much prefer to use muslin (fabric) strips when working on the bikini area. I find it folds into the genital area much easier and seems gentler on the skin. Some people prefer to use paper strips and that is fine as it's all down to personal preference.

When waxing the bikini area on a male or female, there is no need to use long waxing strips. Keep your strips around 5" long. If your strip is around 12" long, like it would be if you were doing a leg or back wax you will have lots of waste and not have as much control as you would do if it was shorter. When the strip is shorter you are able to remove the strip with perfect parallel control. When it is this short you will still be able to have at least 1/3 of the strip free to use as your clean fold, to hold onto when removing the strip.

Glide your hand over the strip towards the hair growth, avoiding rubbing up and down with your hand like you are expecting a genie to appear. Going back and forth is unnecessary and can cause the hair under the strip to weaken and break off. Ever removed a strip before and seen broken hair at the surface? This occurs because of one or two things: Either you rubbed the strip too much, causing the hair to weaken and break off, or when you pulled the strip off, you lifted it *away* from the body, flicking it practically across the room and are left to peel it off the ceiling or the wall opposite to you.

Incidentally, the only time that I do rub the strip like I am expecting a genie to appear, is when I wax the top of my clients feet, during a leg wax. A lot of the time the strip is removed and the wax sticks to the feet because they are cold. I rub the strip to warm the feet up a bit to make it easier to remove. If this still doesn't work, I tuck my gloved fingers under the edge of wax and remove the strip and wax that way, to help ease it from the feet instead. Or I get them to wear socks to keep them warm until I am ready to wax that area.

So, once you have applied the strip and glided your hand across it towards the direction of the hair growth, remove the strip as *parallel* (close) to the skin as possible. As you do this, your wrist should cause a flicking motion or a punching out of the hand. When waxing any part of the body using soft wax, you always keep the strip as close as possible to the skin when removing it. Do this and watch those fat bulbous roots appear on the strip which is what you want. Show your client, frame the darn thing, pat yourself on the back and know that those suckers have come out from their hiding place. When the strip and hair from the patch you have just worked on has been removed, apply firm pressure to the area to relieve some of the *sting*.

You don't need to use a new strip each time, but once the strip has become quite thick with wax, dispose of it and use a new one. Too much wax sitting on the wax strip might save you some money as you won't be going through lots of them, but it doesn't always grip the hair as well as it should do if it is caked with wax residue.

Talk with your client. Try to get to know her by asking questions about her family, hobbies, etc. It keeps their mind distracted and it builds trust also if you show an interest. Ask her what she does for a living and if she lives locally. If you don't get much of a response and she seems reluctant to talk, pay attention to this. She may be shy or she may not want to answer your questions, so don't take it personally.

If she is unresponsive, then quit the chatting, read her body language and just work in silence if that is what you think she needs. Don't take this as a cue for you to start talking about *your* life or *your* latest boyfriend/girlfriend break up. There is nothing worse than a technician who keeps on waffling non-stop about herself and her life... drama, drama, drama. Keep it for those who may want to listen outside of work, but don't bring it into your client's space.

Our clients have personal lives and we don't always know what is happening in their life. They may come to your salon as an escape and a getaway from their hectic, stressed life. Make their experience a pleasant one without them feeling the burden of having to listen to you! This doesn't just apply in the waxing room, but should be a genuine rule of thumb in the service industry, period.

She may not want to make small talk or listen to small talk, but you still need to speak to her as you are informing her each time with what direction you need her hands. She doesn't understand the waxing pattern or your pattern of waxing; she needs to know what her job is during the process.

A Bit about Hair Growth Stages

Without boring you about the anatomy of the hair cycles, I will keep this brief. It is worth you knowing the basics, so you and your client can understand why they may get re-growth in a couple of days after their wax. Hair, that starts to grow back immediately following a wax is not hair that was waxed today, but hair that was just underneath the surface of the skin that you couldn't necessarily see.

It always confused me in beauty school when I was given too many scientific terms associated with hair and it's growth stages, hence the reason I am keeping it simple and trying to get the message across in simple to understand terminology without you falling asleep and drooling at the mouth from boredom.

In an ideal world of waxing and what I picked up in beauty school was that clients should begin their appointments: On day one, then on day fifteen and then again on day thirty for five months. They then start their waxing appointments around the fifth month on a monthly basis. As they approach the seventh month, repeat the one day, fifteenth day, and the thirtieth day process again for one month, and then back to monthly appointments.

Confused? As I said, this is in an ideal world and we all know how difficult it can be at times to get our clients to commit to such a schedule and can also be costly for them. But, if you can get them to follow this routine, then it is even better for their hair growth patterns and will produce better results.

Try it on yourself at home and see if you like it, it makes it easier to 'sell' this idea to your clients and helps you articulate it better to them when you educate them on their own hair growth patterns. Practice what you preach and experience this method yourself to understand the difference it makes when doing it this way.

Hair has three growth cycles:

Anagen (hair bulbs are found nestled in the subcutaneous fat)
Catagen (hair bulbs are found in the dermis)
Telogen (hair bulbs are found in the upper dermis)

During the three stages of hair growth, the bulb is found in different positions as you can see above.

Anagen: This is the active/growing phase and can last for at least three weeks. The cells are dividing rapidly as they sit in the subcutaneous fat, way down deep where we cannot see it. The amount of time it stays in this phase is generally genetically determined. Approximately 85% of all hairs are in the growing phase at this time.

Catagen: This hair is getting ready to shed as it is approaching the dermis and is coming towards the end of the hair growth. It is during this stage that the hair shrinks. Maybe it doesn't want to see daylight and starts to whither away? A bit like me on a Monday morning I suppose!

Telogen: The hair is now resting and is a dead, fully keratinized hair. This is the hair that we see and quite obviously doesn't like daylight as it dies before it get's to this stage! At the end of this phase if the old hair has not already been shed, the new hair pushes it out and the hair growth cycle starts all over again.

Tip 1: What to Do If the Hair Is A Bit Short

Ideally a client should wait at least two to three weeks since shaving, or waxing before her next appointment as the hair is usually not long enough for the wax to grab hold of. But sometimes, a client may come in and her hair is slightly too short in just some places and you don't think the wax will remove all of it. To understand this a little bit more refer back to the previous chapter on hair growth stages.

What I was trained to do during my 2,000 hours of training in the U.K. by my wonderful teacher, was to apply the wax *against* the hair growth. Then, using the same spatula so as not to apply it too thickly, immediately apply the wax *towards* the hair growth. Apply the muslin strip as normal, glide the hand towards the hair growth and remove the strip parallel to the skin as usual. In this way, the motion with the wax on the stick is back and forth.

No double dipping has occurred; it simply means that wax has been applied in two different directions to coat both sides of the hair. The final application of wax is applied towards the hair growth so the hair doesn't just break off at the surface of the skin upon removal which is pointless during waxing. It is also one of the main reasons why ingrown hairs occur.

Remember, no genie rubbing against the strip; a firm glide is sufficient! This method of waxing ***against*** the hair growth is only used when the hairs are teeny tiny and the goal is to remove them without relying on tweezers.

Pre-warn the client that the tiny hairs might be an issue to remove but that you have a technique up your sleeve to help shift the buggers out of their hiding place. Again, sharing this with her will make you more memorable in her eyes, and she will have the confidence that you can rectify problems, come up with a Plan B, and that you put the extra time into her care. This shows professionalism.

Even though the hairs might have been double-sided with wax and you removed the strip correctly, they still might not want to budge. This is when the tweezers have to come out (which I hate). Most clients would prefer to have their bottom impaled by a cactus rather then experience having their nether regions tweezed!

Any technician who spends more time with the tweezers in her hand than the wax needs to re-train or find a job on a farm, plucking chickens. So, if you think that you are one of those secret hair tweezers, keep reading this book, get some more training, or ask for help from your work colleagues. Any successful person is always willing to help others out also. We become successful by helping others to be successful too. It's just plain good karma!

A beauty school teacher of mine in England once used

to stand with her hands on her hips in Miss Bossy Boots stance and say "We tweeze clients and pluck chickens – do not use the term 'pluck' during my class"!

Let me also note that when our client is in our hands on our waxing bed and her hair is too short, too coarse, too long or just unruly – we never, under any circumstances make her feel bad about that. Verbalizing your frustrations at how coarse her hair is, making comments to her such as "Jeez you have strong pubic hair genes lady" or "Oh, my goodness, you are getting all sweaty, do you sweat like this often?" I have heard these comments being used before on clients from students who thought that they were just being nice by sharing their frustrations with the trembling client! I have had to pull them outside for a nice little chat to tell them to zip their comments. Never make your client feel bad about anything that might potentially be going wrong in your room. Your demeanour and professionalism should stay the same no matter what is going on.

If you had a co-worker that was more skilled than what you were – it would be better to say to the client "I am going to go and get Sophie right now, as she is highly experienced in this hair type and will help me get this wax off in a jiffy".

It is better to share the workload with a co-worker that can help you as you will learn by it and the client will leave much happier. The client will understand that Sophie has stepped in to help, because you still have your training wheels on – but she is less likely to understand if you keep on trying and making her feel like it is her problem.

Tip 2: Hair Growth Patterns Down Under

A general rule of thumb, which is not set in stone but is usually pretty accurate, is what I like to refer to as the North, East, South, West factor. Take a look at your own Lady Garden and look at the hair growth. From the pubic bone area, the hair tends to be heading south even though it is in the north sector of the nether regions. Underneath your Lady Garden up the lip/labia, it tends to grow inwards east or west, depending on whether we are looking at the right lip or the left lip.

From the bum hole and some of the labia, it is in the south sector but is growing up to the north. As I said, this isn't set in stone, but, as a guideline, keep it in mind so you get your speed and pattern down a bit better and observe the hair growth as you go.

So, working from the top of the pubic area, I like to work in sections. The side that I am working on around her pubic area and thigh area, I have her angle her leg in a V position so that her heel is parallel to her knee across from her straightened leg. This makes the skin tighter whilst working around it and applying wax. I work around the area, moving towards her thigh and bikini line section.

If she is a pretty toned client with good muscle structure, I can pull the skin taut myself when applying wax and removing it. With the larger built client, who may have more folds or just looser skin around her body, I always get her to hold the skin taut and pull it tightly. I guide her hands as to where I want them and kindly tell her what I would like her to do for me and why. This just simply makes your job easier and it makes it less painful for her and it also avoids bruising.

I then come down towards the thigh area and, wanting to remove some hairs around this area going towards her lady bits, I come across the beast called the *tendon*! I am sure some of you, during your training at beauty school, caused a bruise whilst waxing and was left wondering what the heck you did wrong! Or, you had a bikini wax once yourself and you came out with what resembled a hickey or a love bite on your inner thigh! Try explaining that one to your partner! The tendon is the sensitive structure on the inside of the thigh, which is extremely sensitive and bruises very easily. I will go into how to wax around the tendon in the next chapter.

Once you have finished working from the top of the bikini and around the side, thigh and tendon area, repeat the process on the other side. Get your client to hold her leg in the V position again on the side that you are working on and keep getting her to hold the thigh area or her belly area taut to help you in the process.

Once the area around the top is hair free, there should be a little patch of hair around the pubic bone about an inch in diameter that you have left. I remove this hair with hard wax (stripless wax) as this area is very sensitive for most clients as the hair is denser. This area where the hair is denser is also more prone to breakage. Dust more powder over this area if there are no traces of powder there and with the client pulling her skin ever so slightly upwards apply the hard wax very firmly by *pressing* it into the skin in a figure of eight and remove it efficiently and as close to the skin as possible against the hair growth.

Think of your own pubic bone if you are a female reading this and you have had a full Brazilian wax before. This area is super sensitive *for most people*. It hurts way more than having the labia done, so be conscious of this area and be sensitive to her needs. But don't be too sensitive and squeamish from you're own personal experiences as this will show and you will be hesitant to pull the wax off!!

Tip 3: Bruises/
Hickey Prevention

It's important to pay special attention to the tendon area at all times when waxing and to keep the client's leg in its comfortable V section. The wax is applied down the thigh as the hair in this area tends to grow downward (Think N, E, S, and W!). Apply the wax thinly over that area, keeping the skin taut as you would do normally. Then, apply the strip to the area and, with your other free hand that is keeping the skin taut prior to removing the strip you, tuck a couple of fingers UNDER the tendon.

Pull the strip parallel to the skin, keeping the skin firm but gently with your fingers pressed UNDER the tendon while releasing the strip. Do this properly each time and no bruising will take place. Keep practicing and feeling around under your own tendon, find that little groove section where you can press into it. This area tends not to hurt when pressed underneath, but it does bruise easily if left exposed with no grip protection when a strip of wax is being pulled from it. Always keep the wax application as thin as possible also. If it is too thick, it takes extra work on the skin to remove it, which can also aid in bruising. When using this method, the same applies if you were using hard wax in this area too.

Bruising looks unsightly and shouldn't happen. If it does happen (as accidents can and do happen) explain and apologize to the client immediately that this has occurred. Most of the time, they are okay with it. They may not be over the moon and doing cartwheels naked around your room in excitement because they are leaving with a hickey, but, if you are polite enough and have acknowledged it whilst sweetly saying 'sorry,' then you may be forgiven. If you send them out of the door without so much as an apology, they will be left thinking this is a normal part of the service and chances are, you won't be seeing them again.

I have another story to share with you. During a female Brazilian waxing service, I didn't pay enough attention to this area. Chatting away to my client like I had verbal diarrhoea, I overlooked the necessity to pay extra attention around that area. I was fresh out of beauty school and wanted to cry when I discovered what happened. I got all hot and flustered. I wanted to flee from the room, grab my stuff, and get the heck out of there never to be seen again apart from on the back of a milk carton or under the missing person's section!

My mouth became as dry as a bone and I seriously froze on the spot as that bruise appeared instantly on the surface of the skin like an illuminated light bulb, blinking at me. I was left rooted to the floor, hoping just by some miracle it would disappear or that I would just disappear. I very humbly said, "I am so sorry, but I think when I removed the strip of wax, my pressure must not have been as firm as it *should* have been and it has caused a bruise around your bikini line."

I wasn't met with a smack in the face, but just greeted by a little face from my client, peering between her legs into the bikini area to examine the goods left behind. Both times this has happened to me (you would think I learned the first time!) both clients were 'fine' with it and, yes, I did see them again. Luckily this didn't happen to them again with me and they did become loyal clients after that.

I have to tell you that the first time it happened, I was fresh out of school and my knowledge of the waxing world was a bit vague. The second time it happened, I was overly confident -- cocky you could maybe say -- and was chatting too much. That is when the mishaps occur just as frequently as the times when your knowledge is vague. I knew if I had just sent them home, all waxed and bruised up without me apologizing, they would not have returned to me. Admitting you are wrong or that you have made a mistake is very difficult for some technicians or just people in general, but it's crucial to have excellent customer service when working in the service industry. It means that you have to be pretty humble and apologetic in your approach.

So, try to be humble and offer brilliant customer service when dealing with clients regardless of whether they are there for waxing or other services in your salon or spa. It calls for good etiquette and gets you more recognition in the long term. At the end of the day, who doesn't like to be treated fairly?

Let's recap. Keep the fingers under the tendon to avoid bruising around the upper thigh and always hold the skin taut when applying wax and removing wax. Doing this will always prevent bruising.

Incidentally if a client is on blood thinners, takes aspirin daily, or is vitamin deficient, then no matter what you do to prevent bruises during waxing they may still be more prone.

A superior man is modest in his speech,
but exceeds in his actions.
Confucius

Tip 4 : No Double Dipping

Never double dip! By this I mean that if you have stuck the spatula into the wax pot, then applied it to the area/skin to be waxed, the stick should be thrown away in the trash can immediately. Imagine waxing every client with just one stick and you kept double dipping? The tin of wax would have traces of blood, pubic hair, and faeces (especially if the client didn't clean up properly!!). It would be a breeding ground for bacteria, which is extremely unsanitary and not fair on the clients. If you use small individual pots of wax for one client and one client only and throw the remains away, then, by all means, use just one stick. But, most tins come in standard sizes, and the waste and cost of throwing several wax tins away each day would be far more than the waste and cost of using lots of sticks.

Wax doesn't heat up to a high enough temperature to 'kill' any bacteria. This is a myth, so please don't be fooled into believing this. If anything, since it is kept at a warm temperature, it is more likely to be a perfect breeding ground for germs to fester and multiply. Germs love warm places! Sticks are inexpensive and it doesn't eat away at your profits. Increase your prices by a couple of dollars if it is a big financial concern to you and inform clients as to why your prices are slightly higher.

I would also strongly suggest that you place a sign in your room as well as on your menu or website, informing them that your policy is "no double dipping." Not all salons place signs as they just take it for granted clients know. I think this adds that *extra* uniqueness to your services and business. Some clients wouldn't even think that this was an issue anyway as they may have been informed in the past by a previous aesthetician that the heat of the wax kills germs.

To save a bit of money on the sticks as you do go through a lot of them with body waxing, snap your sticks in half so you have two sticks for the price of one! I personally find the length of the half sticks not long enough though. I prefer a larger handle so I have less chance of getting wax on my gloves. As such, I am happy to just go through a lot of them, but if the waste is of concern to you, then you can try this method.

When I have dipped into the wax with one end of the stick and removed the hair, I then turn the stick around and, with one of the old muslin strips that I have used; I wrap it around the soiled end. I then use the clean side of the muslin as a handle and the other end of the clean spatula to dip into the wax for the next application.

Some may point out that my gloved hands were on this stick prior to it touching the skin. In fact, my hands are on all the products that touch the client. Unless the State Board requires that I work in a NASA spacesuit, with mask and goggles, and spray myself and my client down every five minutes with anti-bacterial spray, then my method is what I shall do. I never double dip, and the used strip wrapped as a handle doesn't come into contact with the wax in the pot either.

It is clean and efficient. Even though money isn't necessarily or shouldn't be a big factor, the waste is really the bigger issue for me. I hate waste of any description and like to keep things recycled as much as possible. I also like to be as sanitary as possible, but I do draw the line at neurotic behaviour!

I will go into 'when it is ok to double dip' in the next chapter, if you still disagree with using hundreds of spatulas.

There are some fantastic waxing educators out there that don't follow this theory and have their own reasons for why it is ok to double dip. I will never criticize what they do or how they do it as that is not my style and it has never been proven from my research that it actually does cause cross contamination. This book is written so that I can share with you what I prefer to do and what I would like to receive if I was on the other end of the waxing service.

Whispering in your ear incidentally, to help you save some pennies – it might be worth you checking out your local arts and crafts store. A lot of these stores sell the wooden sticks/spatulas in all different sizes and it can work out much cheaper than purchasing them from your beauty supply store. My store has some great ones that have a handle with a spoon like end on them. I like to use these when I am working on a small area that is difficult to get into.

Tip 5: When it's Okay to Double Dip

Some technicians love to get their speed up so much so that they can see as many clients a day as possible. These are the technicians who find using new sticks instead of double dipping important but find that it can also be a bit time wasting. So, this is why I mention this method to you.

The method that I am suggesting may also be too time consuming unless you have a large four-heat wax heater since you do have to allow for each new fill of wax pellets to heat up. But, since the level of wax in the tin is low enough for only using on one client, it should heat up pretty quickly. If you can determine how much wax you will need for each client, this should work. And, I am sure over time and with lots of experience you will get some indication as to how much wax you use for each client. If a client is a regular of yours and you know what type of wax you use for them, then this can be heating up prior to their arrival, so you are not twiddling your thumbs waiting for their personal wax tin to heat up.

One idea is to buy wax pellets, which are little beads of wax that come in a jar or bags. If you keep some empty wax tins around, you can place an empty wax tin in your heater before each new client and fill it with as many beads you think you may need for just that *one* client. If that wax is to be used on just that one client alone then double dip to your heart's content. If storage space is an issue in your salon, having lots of personalized tins around might not be a good option.

Because the level of wax in the tin will be pretty low, please ensure, when heating it, that you allow for the low level of wax. By this I mean that if you keep it at the same temperature as you do for a full tin of wax, you may find it's too hot and you will need to wait for it to cool down. Remember, runny wax that drips very quickly in a steady stream off a spatula is too hot!

Just throw the tin away when you have finished waxing your client and use a new tin for each new client. Or, if you prefer, you can line a tin with foil and, when the wax has all gone, remove the foil and replace it with new foil in the tin for the next client. This way you are again avoiding waste and cutting down on cost.

Applying Hard Wax

Most of you are probably aware already from beauty school and prior training in waxing at your salon that hard wax is thicker in consistency and application and is removed without paper strips or muslin strips. Hard wax is fantastic for sensitive areas of the body, such as bikini areas, eyebrows, lips, etc. The reason for this is that hard wax, once applied correctly and at the right temperature, has less contact with the skin than soft wax due to its shrink wrap capabilities around the hair.

I mentioned earlier that I am not an advocate for using soft wax for Brazilians. I always use hard wax on the labia. I never use soft wax on this area as I find the skin is too sensitive and can be looser on some clients than others. I do believe there are some technicians that do use soft wax in this area and they find it works for them and that is ok, if they are doing it correctly.

So, unless your intention is to make handbags out of labia skin, stick to using hard wax – especially if you are still in training!

Hard wax as discussed earlier is much thicker in consistency than soft wax. When applying hard wax anywhere on the body a much firmer pressure is required. As you apply the wax you are actually 'pressing' it down as if you are 'pushing' it into the skin coating the base of the hair snugly. Don't be afraid to press down as firm pressure when applying hard wax is the best way to get a great, clean result. By all means ask your client if the pressure is ok.

If you pull the skin around your elbow, it really doesn't hurt. Try it. Pulling the skin on the labia using your fingertips and not your nails doesn't hurt either and feels similar to the pressure when pulling on elbow skin. It is probably questionable as to whether it hurts or not if your fingernails resemble Freddie Krueger. If that is the case, keep them short!

I like my client to position her leg in the V position as described earlier or have her spread both legs slightly apart like a frog with heels touching heels. Hopefully she hasn't brought Aunt Flow with her, but if she insists on bringing her with her, just get her to tuck the tampon string inside of herself, so you don't have to deal with it!

Sometimes the appointment could have been made weeks prior and Aunt Flow came unannounced and the client still required the service because she was going on a vacation. This happens. We understand being female, that an unannounced seven day guest can arrive days earlier than expected, so don't make a big deal out of it.

As discussed earlier some people like to use a tiny amount of oil prior to the skin before waxing. Depending on the skin and the client's hair, I either use oil or powder. Sometimes I like to use powder more as it shows up the difficult to see hairs, which helps me! I prefer to powder up the labia, so that she has an easier grip on the skin, especially if she is assisting.

The skin on the labia is loose. On some clients it can be very loose. When it is very loose I like her to help me with keeping it taut. With her leg positioned in a V or like a frog, I apply the hard wax going towards the direction of the hair growth in sections pressing the wax firmly as if I am pushing it into the skin. Once the wax has been applied a slight sprinkling of powder can be applied over the applied wax or a clean spatula can be placed *'between'* both of her labia lips.

I want you to place a clean spatula lengthways/horizontal into your mouth right now so it prevents both of your lips from touching (as if you were blotting your lipstick with the spatula or how a dog carries a large stick in its mouth)

This is the position your spatula will be in, when placed between both lips down below. Placing the spatula between her lips down below will prevent the wax from sticking to the opposite lip that we haven't worked on yet.

We does this because once that wax is dry and ready to remove, if traces of wax are sticking to pubic hair on the opposite lip that isn't prepped ready for waxing, it pulls at the hair on the opposite lip causing discomfort to our clients.

If your room is bigger than a postage stamp (and I hope it is bigger, because I know that feeling of trying to work around a room the size of a broom cupboard) try to work your way around the bed applying and removing the wax, until you find the stance that works for *you*! When I teach classes I always tell the students to work from different sides of the bed until you figure out what makes your life easier.

Sometimes if my client isn't heavy set, I get her to raise her hips off the bed slightly, so I have more room to remove the wax. If you feel you are left with very little space to remove this section of wax, you have a tendency to 'flick' the wax off, instead of removing it parallel as you are conscious of the bed getting in the way of your hand motion. When we flick wax off as opposed to removing it parallel, it doesn't make for a clean finish, it breaks the hair off, leaving traces of stubble behind. This can also happen if our body position is clumsy and not comfortable. I go into different methods of hard wax removal later.

When applying wax onto the labia area, if your client is in good shape and is pretty flexible, get her to lift her knee *outward* slightly and up towards her chest area. If she is lucky enough to have large boobies, get her to place her upward positioned leg/knee to the side of her boob as if she is trying to tuck it under her armpit. With her leg positioned slightly outwards it gives you more room and you can get in there much easier than if her inner thigh is pressing against her labia. She can hold onto her knees until you have finished working on this side and are ready to move onto the next side.

Having her in this position keeps the labia pretty taut, making application and removal of wax much easier. Of course you still need to pull the skin taut yourself when you are applying and removing the wax. It's not just a case of stand back, stick your spatula over the labia with an outstretched arm and gently waft it around in a tickle motion. *Get in there.* Don't be afraid to push and firmly apply the wax using pressure, covering as much of an area as confidently possible.

You will pick up speed as you become more confident, so in the meantime, just do it in smaller sections and remove a section at a time when it is dry. I go into speed a few chapters on.

Some aestheticians like to get their clients into the cannonball pose and have them bring *both* legs up to their chest at the same time as described above. When I have been waxed this way it doesn't bother me and I have no inhibitions regarding getting *myself* into this position. But, for some reason, I don't get too many clients who are willing to do this easily for me. No matter how *matter of fact* I am with them about getting into this position, I sense tension from the clients and it doesn't work for me. I have no idea what other technicians do, to get their clients willingly into the cannonball pose, but 'kudos' on them is all I can say. Maybe *they* can share their tips with me one day! One aesthetician I met used to pat her clients on the bottom and boss them into positioning themselves this way. I tried it. It didn't work. I came across like a pervert (or so I thought anyway!) So I prefer to work on clients using the above method.

Also, always think of her under carriage *down under* as being pretty hot... as in: Australia is a pretty hot place to live and is known as "Down Under". Down under in my terms is our under carriage. When we apply hard wax down under, on a male or female the body temperature is hotter than it is up top. This area will take the wax a slightly longer time to set hard than it will on top. You may have found that this is why sometimes when you have tried to remove hard wax from down in her under carriage that, it isn't quite set properly and strings out in the centre, coating your gloved hands with gooey wax. A bit like a brownie consistency where it is gooey in the centre and hard on the outside!

Hard wax with its shrink wrap ability sticks to the hair and not to the skin per se. The beauty of using this wax is that it can be applied in the same area more than once.

I am not saying to keep going over and over the same area hundreds of times, but you have much less chance of burning or lifting the skin than if you did this with soft wax. I do try to avoid applying even hard wax over the same area twice, *especially on the labia*. I just hope my application and correct method of removal is sufficient enough the first time to avoid going over the same area a second time.

But generally, hard wax is pretty much safe to wax over the same area more than once. This is true except if the temperature is way too hot and you burn the living daylights out of her. I am sure this won't happen as we have already discussed the correct consistency and temperature of the wax prior to applying it to the skin.

If you do happen to go over the same area more than once

with the hard wax, due to the skin's sensitivity at *already* receiving wax in this area, the temperature of the wax applied should be cooler, so as not to alert your client with the increase of heat or to burn her.

Reach into the tin with your clean spatula taking the wax from the top without scraping the barrel at the bottom and then keep the wax on the spatula a bit longer, to allow it to cool, before applying it. I have seen some technicians blow the wax like they are spoon feeding their child – there is something about blowing on a waxing spatula that I just find unprofessional!

So, next I will share with you the technique that has always worked well for me. This way, you can try it and see if you like it too. You may want to stick with the regular rule of always applying hard wax towards the hair growth. Again, it's whatever works for you.

Tip 6: Another Way of Applying Hard Wax

I have been taught a few different ways of how to apply hard wax. I was taught my favourite way while I was in beauty school in England. I have also heard from a couple of people that wax should never be applied by fudging or by double-siding the hair due to breakage. I have *never* found this to be the case and I consistently get good results doing it this way.

At this point, hopefully, she still has some dusted powder or a tiny bit of oil around her bits. If she doesn't, apply a little bit more to protect the skin. Again, using a clean spatula so no double dipping occurs, plunge the spatula into the tin from the side, making sure you have a nice fair amount on the end of the spatula like a big garlic bulb.

Sometimes, when pulling the spatula away from the tin with the wax attached to the end, there are 'stringy' bits of wax attached to it. I have seen some aestheticians keep pulling the spatula away from the tin to help detach the strings, but then they spun themselves around in circles or, even worse, circle the spatula above their head trying to get rid of the stringy wax. The result is that they then became like a cocoon of wax where it sticks to their clothes, the equipment, the walls and even their shoes!

If you have done this, I am sure you will be smiling right now as you know exactly what I am talking about! With the spatula and blob of wax attached to the end, just waft it back and forth in the tin very close to the heat of the wax without actually touching the wax in the tin, and this will break the string free for you. Incidentally, when you have applied the hard wax onto the body, waft the spatula back and forth, close to the wax application also. The heat from the wax will prevent strings.

The wax is then applied *firmly* in a figure of eight. Apply the wax going down the hair in a section *towards* the hair growth, then back up again and around and up the hair *against* the hair growth, then completing the circuit again by going back *towards* the hair growth. In this way, you are forming a figure eight in one of your sections, which will be about 1 ½" - 2" in width and length. What this does is coat the hair on both sides.

When you firmly apply the hard wax, you should always try to keep the edges of the wax around the figure eight in an even consistency. When some of the edges are too thin, as they dry, they then become brittle. When pulled off the skin, this tends to leave annoying traces of hard wax. Leave the wax to dry for a couple of minutes and whilst you are doing this, you can prepare your hard wax removal handle.

I can explain another way of applying the hard wax if you are not happy with the figure eight method. Basically, the wax is applied using a clean spatula again onto the hair in the direction of the hair growth just the same as applying soft wax. Again, keep the edges the same thickness so it doesn't get too thin. A lip can be formed or you can use another method of removal using a handle of your choice. The wax is applied pushing it into the skin in the direction of hair growth and removed against it. It is removed by keeping it as close to the skin as possible just like when waxing with soft wax.

This is quite simple with no fuss and the best part of all is that you don't need to be a rocket scientist to figure it out. But, for some reason I just find this way doesn't get as *clean* a result as what I would like hence the reason I prefer the figure eight method. However, you may love to apply it this way and want to stick with it. Whatever works for you safely and for your client is the way you should go and the way you should stick to. Be comfortable, but be safe.

Now some clients have hair that is growing inside the labia. This area is extremely sensitive and the skin is very thin here.

Pull one of her lips slightly apart and she can assist you by pulling the other lip away for you if that helps. When I apply powder to this inner labia area, I always place a clean spatula lengthwise to protect her Lady Garden "opening" from being exposed to powder. Powder entering the Lady Garden itself can be very irritating and can most certainly cause an irritation that can potentially lead to an infection from scratching. So protect her opening from anything going into it.

I keep this area of waxing to a minimum and take extra care that wax isn't going into the darkness of the abyss and where there is no hair.

Girls, lets talk about our lovely Lady Gardens: Shut your bathroom door, get out a mirror and look at your privates. Inside the Labia Garden is a shiny wall, it is slightly more red in color than the outer labia and very rarely does it have hair growing out of it. If for some reason your client does have hair growing out of this area and she wants it removing DON'T DO IT! This area is very thin and this area is the area that most nurses in the ER see disastrous results from bikini waxing services that have gone wrong. If your client is adamant that you dig totally in her Garden with your lawn mower, get out your tweezers and tweeze the very few hairs that will be there. Waxing over shiny skin inside the Garden is dangerous, please don't do it.

Tip 7: Removing Hard Wax

Using a clean spatula, dip into the tin, remove a blob of wax from the side about the size of a quarter coin, and blob the wax onto the *inside* of *your* arm where there is no hair. To speed up the drying process, sprinkle some powder over it and dab it lightly. *Sprinkling powder onto hard wax speeds up the drying time.*

When the waxed figure of eight on the client is firm to the touch and ready to remove, you can then take the dried blob that is sitting on the inside of your arm and, with the shiny side of the wax (the wax that is not touching your skin), form a tab onto the figure eight to work as your handle. Place the wax from the inside of your arm onto the wax where you want to lift it from and remove the wax from your client this way. Think shiny side to shiny side.

Lift the wax from the hair against the hair growth, using your wax handle to remove it. The reason I use a handle is to prevent picking at the edges of the wax, which can sometimes cause more discomfort than the wax removal itself. So, don't pick at the edges to remove it, use a handle or leave a larger blob of wax for easy removal as explained below.

Picking at the edges of the wax bugs the "geebies" out of clients and feels very irritating, inevitably also picking at their skin.

Removing hard wax is the same principle as removing soft wax. Pull it away from the hair/skin as parallel to the body as possible to prevent leaving traces of hair or breaking it off at the surface.

Another way of removing hard wax is by leaving a much thicker blob of wax at the point where you know you want to remove the wax from. This is called 'forming a lip.' The area left will be thicker with a slight lip and this can be used as your handle when removing the wax to avoid any picking.

Tip 8: Caterpillar trail

Another way of removing the hard wax is to create what I call a Caterpillar trail. This is an advanced method that is used once your technique is up to speed and you are pretty confident with your waxing services. Now your brain might be buzzing around like a fly in a shoe box taunted by the different removal methods, but they are all actually good tips to have up your sleeve and make your business much more fun and effective.

So, now she has a figure eight of wax stuck to her under carriage and you are waiting for it to dry. This isn't the only hair around her labia so once you have applied this section with hard wax go onto another section and do the same thing again. This can be done three or four times in different sections around the area, coating different sections of hair. Remember "Down Under" is warmer, so the drying time will be longer.

When you look at her nether regions, you will see that she has patches of wax all over her in different places. This method is used in speed waxing and, again, I wouldn't do this method until you are pretty confident with your technique. You also have to have a pretty good memory as to which section you applied wax too first, and which direction the hair is growing in, underneath it.

With practice and knowing your (N, E, S, W) rule of thumb, it starts to become second nature. Let's say for argument sake you have four sections of wax scattered around her Garden. The first section by now will be pretty dry so you remove this first section (by using a handle of your choice). With the shiny side of the wax that you have *just* removed, attach it to section number two and pull the second section off using the first blob of wax as your handle. Keep, using these as your wax handles until all waxed sections have been removed. It makes the removal process much quicker and you avoid picking at the wax. Again, think shiny side to shiny side.

Tip 9: Positions

Everything above is super smooth -- no hickies, no irritated skin, and a happy smiley client. Now it's time to get the client to turn over so you can wax her bum crack.

There are four different ways that I have been taught how to do this. Anatomy of the client does play a big part in how we wax this area as does the client's personality.

Each of the four ways is explained below. You can be the judge of what you like the best and I will share with you what I do prefer and why.

1. **The cannonball position**
   With your client lying on her back, ask her to bring her knees up to her chest, spreading her legs slightly as she does this. She will resemble a trussed up turkey ready for roasting without the little white caps on her feet! Please note that this is not an easy position for a heavy set client or a pregnant client to get into.

   Once she is in this position, you can get a good view of her bum obviously, but it also forces the area to be waxed to be pulled pretty taut, which makes application and removal easier.

She also has a much higher chance of tooting gas whilst she is in this position and, personally, I don't want to be on the receiving end of it! I am not a lover of this position for my clients, or for myself.

Apply the powder to her exposed area so the powder sticks to the hair and not so much her bum hole. Apply the hard wax in small sections and, once dry, remove the wax. Remember 'Down Under' we are a bit hotter, so it might take longer to dry. The spatula can also be applied to separate the two bum cheeks from sticking together or a slight dusting of powder can be applied over the wax to prevent this from happening.

Strangely enough, most clients tell me that this area is not at all painful, but some clients actually tell me that it feels quite nice to have the warm wax applied here and then removed. I ask no questions about their private life or their fetish that involves hot wax applied to their bum. To each their own is my philosophy. After all, what do I care what they find soothing in the comfort of their own home?!

2. <u>**Doggy Style position**</u>

Get your client to get on all fours on the bed, again with her legs spread slightly apart. You will have to get her to spread one bum cheek apart with one hand whilst balancing on the bed with her other hand to support her. This is not an easy task for an older client or a very, very heavy client. The visual for some aestheticians is also not a good one and will stay inputted in the brain for many months to come!

The bum cheek that is spread apart makes it easy for you to apply the powder and the wax because the skin is taut so it makes it easier. Encourage her to pull tightly to keep the skin as taut as possible. Of course, you can also pull one bum cheek apart, whilst you apply and remove the wax. It's whatever you find the easiest.

3. **Flat Waxley**

Get your client to lie down on the massage bed onto her stomach. Then have her spread both bum cheeks apart as wide as possible to make the application of powder and wax as easy as possible. Prep the skin and apply the wax as normal. This is my favourite position for clients to be in. I feel they have some dignity left and have less chance of tooting gas (which is enough of a reason to prefer this position). It is also a pretty standard easy position for any client regardless of body shape, type, etc.

4. **Side Plank.**

This position is very similar to Flat Waxley but with the client lying on her side. I like this way of doing it also, especially if the client is slightly claustrophobic and doesn't like her face pressed into the bed or massage/facial hole. This is the way that most midwives remove stitches from an episiotomy following child birth. It also allows the client to keep some dignity as they feel less exposed. She will still need to help by pulling her bum cheek slightly apart so that you can get into the area easily with your wax and it will also keep the skin taut, making removal much easier.

Excellence is in the details. Give attention to the details and excellence will come.
Perry Paxton

How is your speed baby?

Of course I am all about the speed as time is money, but I wouldn't say I was the fastest waxer on the block. If you spend an hour on a bikini wax because you are new to the service that is fine. Take your time as speed is not of any importance to you right now. Being thorough and understanding the female anatomy from a waxing standpoint coupled with understanding wax, how it works, the issues that you might come across with the wax (and you will) the positioning and learning to talk all at the same time, all takes time! Don't be hard on yourself if you feel the client is getting bored and has things to do. If she is a non-paying client and she is aware of the fact that you have your training wheels on, then she should show some patience.

For this reason (as we do come across some clients, that are sooo important and have sooo much to do and lack patience in all areas of their lives, but just want a freebie…. scoff, scoff) for the first ten clients you practice on should be friends, co-workers or family members.

Once you have gained a bit of confidence from working on co-workers and friends etc then roll in the non-paying clients and use them as your models until you pick up speed and confidence. Incidentally, your speed will pick up once your confidence has improved. Confidence will only come from practice and making some mistakes along the way. Any aesthetician who tells you that she has never made a mistake or had a bad waxing experience at some point is a lying ninny!

I have been known to do a full leg wax, eyebrow wax, and a full Brazilian in thirty minutes. This is a very rare occurrence for me. Generally when I am waxing, we are chatting, I am becoming much acquainted with the client and I can honestly say we are having a pretty good time!

I am not in it for the speed or to get the fastest bikini waxing certificate nationally. This is of no interest *to me*. The money is juicy and pays the mortgage, but it's also juicy and pays the mortgage when I am taking my time and not stressing myself out.

On average it takes me to do a full Brazilian approximately twenty minutes. This includes stopping from time to time; to chat with the client, maybe change into a less sticky pair of gloves, or to just stop and listen to her by maintaining eye contact, giving her my full attention.

There is no right or wrong way. It is what works best for you and for your client. I have never had a new client, who specified when climbing on the bed, that she had to be out in ten minutes. If I did, her service can be re-scheduled for a day when she is not so busy! If she was a regular client and I knew her body and didn't need to make small talk to get to know her, then this is different. But, I would still tell her to allow herself enough time next time so we can be as thorough as possible without the pressure of being rushed.

Some clients once they have received a super, five minute bikini wax from the salon down the street thought it was fantastic that they were in and out in no time, but even if their next bikini wax took ten minutes longer at a different salon, it wasn't a deal breaker for them.

If you have been waxing professionally for over a year and you are still taking around forty-five minutes to an hour, I would say this is too long. Your speed should be a bit faster. But, and here is the *but*, I have no idea what your financial goals are, what your financial books at your salon look like or what your main objective is within your waxing career, or how your clients even feel about the time length. But, one thing I can say is "if it works for you and for the salon that you are working for, then who am I to tell you to pick up speed?" You may have the highest client retention rate than anybody in your city. If you started to increase your booking schedule by 50% because you decide to install a revolving door in your salon to compete with your competitors creating something that you were just not comfortable doing, simply because you were doing it for all of the wrong reasons, then you are in trouble.

You know your goals, what your objectives are and what you want your finances to look like, so you are the judge of what works best for you. Let's not forget though, that right now we are talking about what *you* want, what works best for *you*. Your client is No 1 and don't forget this! Her safety is your main priority and your retention rate say's a lot about your reputation. Keep your reputation away from the ER!

Some five minute waxers might double dip, they might not be warm and fuzzy, they might not interact and build client relationships, they might not send thank you cards, because they are too busy waxing. They might not take the time out to walk the client out to the door, introducing her to product along the way or to introduce her to another service for another day. I say 'might' because not all five minute speed waxers *are* this way. But if you could take just that bit longer and do all of the above with the client I know from experience what clients prefer and what they like to return back too.

The late client

Ok, I am a Virgo and tardiness is one of my biggest pet peeves! What is it with people that just can't show up for an appointment on time? If you are late for a Doctors visit, you miss it and more often than not you get charged for it. If you don't show up for a Dermatologist's appointment you get charged for it. If you are running late for a Lawyer's appointment, the clock is ticking and you get a hefty bill for time not spent. If you book a table at the busy, trendy restaurant down the street that everybody is talking about and you are late, they give the table away to other trendy, hungry mouths that are getting in on all of the fun, whilst you and your friends are out in the cold, with your noses pressed against the window observing the feast and famine inside!

So, why is there is such a grey area in our industry when it comes to this issue? Some salons charge a percentage to the no show client or they charge the full amount to the client. Some salons don't charge them anything and don't take a credit card upon booking the appointment. I have worked in both environments. The respect you got from the clients and the way it made your tardy or no show clients jump to attention was from the latter. Once they missed an appointment and got charged something for it, they never did it again. Occasionally, a client *might* get her knickers in a twist because they got charged and may never step foot in your door again. I would prefer regular clients who show up and who show up on time knowing that this is our policy, rather than having a handful of clients on my books that day that had reputations of hitting the missing person's list from time to time making me lose money in the process.

When I worked at the salon that didn't charge no-shows or penalize sweetly the late ones I was forever having clients that just swiftly blew their high maintenance selves in from the street without so much as an apology, and still requiring the same time length for the service. That was a tough one and not one I would recommend to anybody. I think it makes salons look desperate and desperate breed's complacency.

People will treat you, however *you* let them!

Now the late client is another concern as you want to get her in and out, so you can make sure that your following client who is most likely on time for her appointment, actually get's into your room at the appointed time. It is not fair on the following client if you make her late, when she has made the effort to get there swiftly.

I once worked in a very, very high end hotel and at this location the client was always, always right. The client is always right in most incidents in the service industry whether we like it or not and we should always make them feel this way. (Unless it involves assault or sexual harassment) For instance we would never tell a client that they are 'wrong'. We might not agree with them or like what they are doing or saying, but we don't tell them that they are 'wrong'. What we were told to sweetly say at the high end hotel I worked at was "Hello, Mrs Fat-ass, we are already twenty minutes into your appointment time, so let's get you back here so we can efficiently begin your service" How can they argue with that? It is important to say this upon greeting them so it prevents them from then saying "Oh, let me just pop into the ladies room". If they are late for an appointment, popping into the ladies room chips another ten minutes into the appointment time, especially if she is Mrs Dithering Knickers! They might, mumble something under their breath about why they are late, but *you* have set the record straight that it has not gone unnoticed that they are late and that you have another punctual client waiting. (Incidentally, we really didn't call our late clients Mrs Fat-ass!!)

If a client is running really late and you just don't think you have time to see her that day, then maybe you can schedule her with another technician who isn't busy, or re-schedule her appointment. Re-scheduling appointments for late clients or no shows should always be done nicely. Again, don't tell them that they are wrong, or that they need to buy a watch, or who the heck do you think you are just waltzing in, in your own merry sweet time? Be empathic, but also be firm as this is your policy.

Most salons have a twenty minute window. After twenty minutes they are classed as a no-show and have to re-schedule. If your client does eventually drag her sorry bum into your salon twenty minutes late and you *don't* have another appointment scheduled, then by all means take this client, but make a point of saying sweetly "It's your lucky day Mrs Pea-Brain, even though you are running behind today I can still take you, because I don't have a conflicting appointment straight after you, as normally under those circumstances we would have to re-schedule your appointment"

It's a bit like dating really! If in the beginning you allow your date to treat you a certain way, without sticking up for yourself, the more they will do it and get away with it! So flex your muscles, know your self worth and know how you want to be treated and watch them flock to your feet!

Client Clean-Up

Check under your magnifying light for any stray hairs that hopefully you didn't miss! If you really have too, get out the tweezers and tweeze away at a few of them. This should not be a big part of the clean up process and with practice and experience; the tweezers shouldn't be used very much.

This is also a time during the clean up process where you will see if (god forbid!) any skin has lifted. What you will see if this has happened is a change in texture on the skin. It will have a *shine* to the skin. This *shine* to the skin is what will scab over and cause discomfort to the client. It is basically new skin and I hope this doesn't happen to you, but if it does, apply a small amount of antiseptic lotion to the area and tell your client apologetically that unfortunately this has happened and that she will need to continue dabbing it to the area once she is home for the next few days. In your early days of waxing especially during the training period you may have this happen, but as your experience grows it will become very infrequent.

Apply a nice Aloe Vera soothing lotion, hydrocortisone lotion, salicylic acid 1% or 2% lotion or any other nice soothing lotion by the company of your choice. Rub the lotion into your gloved hands to warm it up a little bit and to help with the slick. Apply the lotion, rubbing it in gently, but efficiently.

If she has some sticky residue left from waxing, get her to rub around that area to help remove it.

I would not recommend handing her a hot towel at this point to soothe her nether regions as the area is delicate and probably a bit red from the waxing. At this point, a slight amount of redness is perfectly normal. However, red skin and hot towels are not a good combination. Wait for the damp hot towel from your hot towel cabinet to reach a comfortable temperature before applying it to the area to help relieve some irritation and to calm the skin down.

During the clean-up period, this may be a good time (if you have the time on your books) to cross-sell your services. If you noticed whilst you were waxing her that she had hair on her legs or her brows needing shaping, then by all means ask her if this is a concern for her and advise her as to how wonderful you could make them look. If she doesn't have time that day, suggest it for her next visit. Maybe you could suggest that if this is for a special occasion that you *Vajazzle* her Garden before she leaves. I go into what Vajazzling is, later on in the book.

This is also a good time to suggest to her that it is important that she keeps on a schedule as much as possible and become a regular at waxing to maintain the hair growth. If she shaves in between, the hair will grow back coarser; making her next wax feel like it is her first wax and really defeats the object of waxing.

Hair grows back finer the more that you wax it. Some of the follicles die or weaken, causing the hair to grow back slightly sparser and fluffier than if they were to shave or to use depilatory creams. Clients do find that it gets easier with each wax that they have due to this very reason.

Unfortunately it rarely gets to the point of no hair growth as this doesn't happen with waxing! Explaining to them the reasons behind why waxing is so beneficial also helps them to understand why they put themselves through the whole procedure!

Inform her that every four weeks is a good period, but this can vary with each client and can also vary due to different ethnic backgrounds. Some clients may need waxing every six weeks as opposed to four. Or if you want to suggest to her that she follows the *Ideal* waxing procedure as discussed earlier you could do this also.

What your Client
needs to know

There are a couple of things that your client needs to know before she leaves your salon. Advise her to avoid Jacuzzi's, tanning beds, sauna's or steam rooms for at least twenty four hours following a wax. The pores have been opened and are more prone to infection.

Going to the gym *immediately* following a wax is also not advisable, as sweat can cause the skin to break out or become irritated. Remember the yeast infections mentioned earlier in the book? And I would not recommend using a Loofah as explained earlier due to its porous nature and ability to harbour yeast also!

A nice warm tepid shower with nothing too scented or abrasive for twenty four hours is the best way to treat the areas that have been waxed. After twenty four hours, if the skin is not too inflamed and irritated then a good sugar scrub is great to use twice a week to help prevent in grown hairs, followed by a good soothing lotion to keep the skin calm in the nether regions.

I like to tell my clients that their skin has been through some sort of minor trauma and to treat it, just like they would if they had sunburn. After all you wouldn't go rubbing yourself with an abrasive scrub, steaming yourself like a vegetable or tanning your body, if you were already sunburnt!

If this is her first time with waxing or if you are still waxing with your training wheels on and you think she is a bit red and looking sore – tell her to drink lots and lots of water. Drinking lots of water will make her 'pee-pee' less acidic so when she next visits the loo, it won't create a stinging sensation!

Wearing tight fitting jeans is ok if they have had a wax from the waist up, but anything below the waist, then they need to wear loose, comfortable fitting clothes for at least twenty four hours. This helps prevent chaffing of the skin and also helps prevent ingrown hairs!

Some clients may break out regardless of your skill or which wax was used. If this is the case it is best that they come back in to see you so that you can inspect their area of concern and recommend a product to help them with this.

Witch Hazel is a great inexpensive product to use at home if they break out or suffer from any irritation.

A good homemade mix whipped up in the kitchen of aspirin and water is a good topical treatment to use also to help with any irritation. If possible, let them know that breakouts sometimes happen and that *next time* you will use a wax specifically for sensitive skin. If it is their very first wax appointment, then let them know this is very common and it sometimes takes a few sessions for their skin to get used to it.

If this does happen to one of your clients then make a note of it on their client record card: so you can either, ask them about it again the next time that you see them, or phone them to find out how they are doing, if you haven't seen them for a while.

This shows that you took the time to remember that they had an issue with their last waxing appointment and that you care!

How to Remove Ingrown Hairs

Ingrown hairs are very common in the bikini area. They are generally caused by incorrect waxing, or shaving. They are also caused by wearing very tight, synthetic underwear or tight jeans following a wax. When the skin isn't allowed to breathe it sweats and bacteria gets trapped leading to zits and ingrown hairs.

Exfoliating the bikini area twice a week with a nice scrub, helps unclog the pores by removing the dead skin cells surrounding the follicle also.

Using a nice hot compress applied to the area for five minutes will help draw out the gunk making its exit strategy easier. Gently apply pressure either side of the bump where the ingrown hair is to see if this helps. If nothing seems to be coming out, apply your hot compress again and repeat the process.

If you still have no joy, then leave it alone. Too much squeezing can rupture the follicle underneath the skin resulting in an infection, bleeding or scarring.

If you do see the tip of the hair pop out when applying pressure to the area – using your clean, sanitized pointy tweezers remove the hair and then apply a Tea Tree astringent compress to help remove any bacteria. Tea Tree has wonderful properties as its natural agent cures fungus, bacteria and most viruses. It can also be used as a mouthwash diluted with water if you have forgotten your toothbrush!

If it still looks slightly inflamed a touch of high frequency will help reduce the inflammation and help to kill any bacteria that may be present. Even better to help with reducing inflammation and the extraction of an ingrown hair is *Epsom salts.*

Epsom salts are named from a bitter, saline spring at Epsom in Surrey, England. It is not actually a salt but a natural occurring mineral with *amazing* health benefits which contain magnesium and sulphites. These two powerful ingredients help remove ingrown hairs as they are both readily absorbed through the skin improving the absorption of nutrients and aid in flushing out the toxins. The salts when used as a compress alleviate pain and inflammation. It also exfoliates the dead skin cells without causing a stinging sensation. It is a great alternative from using just a regular compress of hot water. Epsom salts are very, very inexpensive and can be found in most pharmacies/chemists. They can be used for a whole variety of ailments and not just for the flushing out of ingrown hairs.

Buy a large, medicine glass bottle and store your labelled salts in there, to use in your salon for cleaning, medicinal purposes or to just look 'fancy'!

Mix 2 tablespoons of Epsom salt into a bowl with 8 oz of distilled water (tap water is ok, but it's preferable to use distilled) Soak your cotton compress into the solution and leave on the infected or ingrown area for a minimum of ten minutes.

Epsom salts rough texture makes it an ideal exfoliator which you can use on yourself at home. Massage handfuls of it over your body during your shower to rid the skin of any dead skin cells and to give you that healthy, happy glow! It can also be mixed in with a cleanser as a facial scrub. Tea Tree can be added to your little mixture too, if you have oily skin.

You can tell your clients about this wonderful alternative to an expensive scrub, but if retail is where you make most of your profits, maybe you can keep this secret to yourself!

I would love to share with you a secret solution (not that it will be a secret anymore!) that I highly recommend for you to retail in your salon and to also use as a take home pressie for your first time clients that might be susceptible to getting ingrown hairs. This company is based in the U.S and has a fantastic solution that I love to use myself after a wax and find that clients enjoy wearing them also.

They are called "Knicker Stickers". They are packaged nicely and are hygienically made from 100% breathable cotton and made in the U.S! They come in two different colors, beige and black. They basically stick into your trousers like a panty liner but without the feeling of wearing a nappy or a pair of old ladies incontinence knickers. *Wearing them in your trousers without your knickers on will leave you feeling foot loose and fancy free, without any tight underwear chaffing along your bikini line. At $7.95 for a pack of seven, I think that is a pretty good deal to either give one away to first time waxing clients or to retail the whole pack of seven, so that she can wear one each day for a week! Their original purpose is to wear them for preventing panty lines, travelling and the whale tail.*

After realising that it actually worked for ingrown hair prevention, I put a whole new spin on them for myself! Does your competition offer this freebie? I bet they don't!

*Please, inform the client that you are sending them home with a "knicker sticker" simply for the reason that it helps reduce the possibility of getting ingrown hairs. Stating this fact will make you sell more of them, when clients understand that it is a benefit to them and **not** because you are a sloppy waxer that has left big globs of wax in her Garden!*

Tip 10: High Frequency

A little device that so many of my male clients love but of course can also be used on a female after waxing is the high frequency machine. Whenever I wax a client's back, chest or bikini and he/she appears to be on the red side or is prone to breaking out, I get out the ole faithful high frequency machine. For some reason this little machine makes men feel ever so loved, more than it does for women!

High frequency kills bacteria, speeds up the healing process, and the current from the high frequency provides an infusion of oxygen molecules into the skin. The high frequency current also produces a cleaning and massaging method. The massage stimulates the blood flow, which helps carry the waste away by the lymphatic system. The client will experience a therapeutic tingling sensation. Inside the little glass mushroom probes are neon and helium. These two gases are what makes the probes look violet or pink in color. The rapid oscillation of the current improves the process of nourishment to the area and can stimulate hair growth. But don't worry about applying high frequency over a freshly waxed area; it is not that effective that hair will start sprouting out immediately like a Chia seed head commercial! Heat is brought to the area which then soothes the nervous system, without providing heat in such a way to the waxed area that will leave the skin more red than usual. It does just the opposite.

It is also nice to use around the brow area if your client is heading back into work after an eyebrow wax. Apply a nice soothing lotion to the area that has been waxed. Then give a nice brow massage applying gentle pressure to the brow bone. Apply some dry gauze and begin to glide the high frequency gently over the area to be treated. The high frequency current is much more stimulating and produces ozone when applied over dry gauze. Again, I inform my clients about this.

It also helps to reduce the redness and again makes them feel that you are taking extra care into their needs. Avoid the eyeballs; just glide it across the brow bone for a minute or so!

If like I mentioned earlier she has some lifted skin (God forbid!) then the high frequency applied over the area with Neosporin® and facial gauze on it will help with the healing process also.

Remember when applying the high frequency machine to keep your finger on the glass mushroom probe until it touches the skin. If you place the glass probe directly to the skin without easing your finger off it when you touch her, it will spark and shock her. It will not shock her as in giving her an electric shock or by hurting her, but it will just startle her as it will feel like a rubber band twanging against her. So, remember, each time you remove the probe or apply the probe, keep the pointer finger on it until contact is made.

Clients really do like it, and it does reduce a lot of the redness and is very beneficial for zits and the prevention of further breakouts, but it is also soothing to the skin due to its oxygenating properties. All these benefits surely help towards increasing your retention rate and tips!

However, those clients who are epileptic, pregnant, have metal implants or who have a pacemaker are not a good candidate for the high frequency machine. So, if you plan on using this machine after waxing, ask your clients if they are or have any of these contraindications.

In normal brain function we have millions of tiny electrical charges that pass from our nerve cells in the brain to the rest of the body. When the brain function is interrupted by unusual bursts of electrical energy (which high frequency produces) a person who is epileptic receiving this may have a reaction, resulting in a seizure.

Pacemaker failures can occur when they are exposed to high voltage electricity. High frequency interferes with their device and can be fatal.

Clients with metal implants, metal braces and a mouth full of dental fillings are also advised not to receive high frequency. Exposure to rapidly changing magnetic fields especially on metal implants can cause parts of the body to heat up. A decisive factor is the conductivity of the metal. Heat that is produced is conducted to the surrounding tissue and in a worst case scenario can cause the surrounding tissue to sustain burns.

Over four million women in the U.S.A give birth every

year and nearly one third of them will have some kind of pregnancy related complication. Epidemiological studies suggest that low energy that is transmitted from a high frequency electromagnetic field may cause biological effects, such as damage to the DNA and changes in oxidative metabolism in the fetus. So to be on the safe side, keep the high frequency machine away from your pregnant clients.

Hopefully I have given you enough serious but important information about high frequency and its benefits coupled with its contraindications. But it's now time to press on to something a bit less technical for my frizzled brain so I can leave the serious electrical jargon to the scientists!

The hair is removed... how about Vajazzling that baby!?

What is Vajazzling some may ask? Vajazzling is a fantastic service that you can get your clients to up grade too from their Brazilian wax. It is very easy to sell this add on service to your clients, and it doesn't take you long to do *and* it's a great way of making additional money. This is a great service to sell to your client if she is going on a honeymoon, vacationing with her love bug or just spending a lovely sexy evening home with her partner.

Once the bikini area has been freshly waxed you can apply nice jewels in the shape of flowers, stars, or butterflies onto her mowed area, or she can design her own. These jewels are referred to as "Vajazzling".

They are applied with self adhesive glue to an area that is dry and free from lotions and they usually last approximately two to three days, if she takes care to not be too rough in this area with washing and rubbing etc or by wearing tight fitting clothing.

After all a girl needs to take care of her diamonds!

They are applied firmly onto the top of the bikini area, just above the pubic bone area and can be adjusted into shape very easily with tweezers. They are becoming quite a hit across the world!

There are a few companies to choose your jewels from on my website and they all have very promising reputations. Let's hope we get more companies producing such wonderful accessories for our lady bits!

You can very easily upgrade her service, give her partner something to be happy about *and* make her feel *secretly* special at the same time.

There is also since writing this book, rumours about 'Pejazzling' becoming popular. I am sure it will be a huge hit, especially with our wonderful, flamboyant gay male clients! Maybe you can encourage your female clients to bring in their male friends to get the Twigs and Berries waxed and have a nice jewelled display in the shape of a guitar or whatever else they might have out there onto his tackle. I bet that is one secret that client won't be sharing with his friends over a beer one night! But his partner will know and it can become their own little secret – (if he buys into it, of course!)

I once heard from a fellow aesthetician that she did a Vajazzling service on a seventy year old lady, who was celebrating her 50th wedding anniversary! I bet her husband nearly died of fright seeing his wife's bare Lady Garden displayed with an English jewelled crown on her lady bits! I hope he made it to their 51st wedding anniversary after that delightful surprise.

Big girls need big diamonds.
Elizabeth Taylor

Sex following a full mowing of the Lady Garden

I don't know of any clients that have ever come back to me, confessing that they had major irritation from sex following a bikini wax.

In an ideal world a person in the medical profession, would advise a client against having sex for at least twenty four hours following a full Brazilian wax.

The hair follicles have been opened and are more prone to infections than normal. The rubbing motion that occurs during a good ole romp in the hay down below can cause some irritation, resulting in the client scratching the skin, which in turn can lead to an infection.

It's one of those comments that might be worth mentioning to your clients in passing, but one that I doubt very much they would take any notice of, especially if she is getting her Garden groomed for a special event and she has some lovely Vajazzling action going on down there also.

If she comes back to you next time, complaining that she was more irritated after her last wax than she usually is, this could be the reason. So pointing it out to her beforehand will help eliminate further discussion and will help prevent you from having to ask her "So, you were more irritated than usual…hmm, did you get all down and dirty that night?" Save the personal information as it's none of your business what she did that night with her freshly mowed Garden!

How is her bum looking?

I am going to briefly discuss with you another 'hot topic' that seems to be taking America by storm. Not sure if the Europeans are rushing out to get their bums all peachy as of yet, but I am sure it will only be a matter of time! So let's get to the bottom of this shall we? (Pun intended!)

Anal bleaching. That's right 'anal bleaching' is not just for the porn industry anymore! More and more people are opting to get their bums bleached. Now before I get hate mail from any readers, wondering why on earth I would be suggesting such a thing let me tell you this has nothing to do with me as I am just the messenger. I know they say *shoot the messenger* but I would prefer you all to play nice in the sand box and just listen to what I have to say.

Both male and females from different ethnic groups sometimes have concerns with how they look down there. Some people have a darker area down there which they are just not happy about. Some don't care and are happy with what they have and some probably have no clue what their bum looks like anyway!

But, for those clients who are just not happy with the color of themselves down below, they now have an option to have it bleached. There are services out there for everybody and as aestheticians we are empathic enough hopefully, to show some care and consideration towards our clients with any concerns that they have.

As we build relationships with our clients, they spill some very personal secrets with us at times and confide in us more than they may with their friends. After all, going out for dinner with friends is not the time to confess over the appetizers that "life is great, apart from the color of my bum hole!"

Because this book covers the topic of waxing the intimate areas and usually involves waxing this area also, it gives me the perfect opportunity to casually mention this to you so that you can discuss this service with your clients if you so choose. If your client is very concerned about this area, he or she may mention it to you in passing. This then gives you the opportunity to suggest that they have it bleached in your salon a few days after their waxing appointment. If you spend time waxing down there, then it should really make no difference to you whether you are waxing the area or bleaching it. Retail some tubes of the cream in your salon and educate your clients on how to use it properly at home.

If your client doesn't mention her darkened bum concerns to you, but you notice this area is much darker than the rest, just merrily in a very matter of fact way, tell her what one of the latest trends is right now. She might bite the bullet and push you for more information. If anything, you will both probably have a giggle out of it! If she doesn't pursue the conversation, you could be treading on dangerous ground, so just change the topic to the weather instead!

I am a big believer in *shock value*. Shock value, 'shocks' and get's people attention. Even if your client is not the slightest bit interested in getting her bum hole bleached, I bet you all the tea in China that she will mention it to at least four people that week that the salon she goes to offers anal bleaching. Those four people that she shares this information with will mention it to other people and your salon name will be one big word-of-mouth machine. They might not all come crashing your door down to get bum bleaching, but they might be curious as to what other new and trendy things you are keeping abreast of.

So keep up to date with new things as much as you can and always check with your State Board of Barbering and Cosmetology that this isn't a salon faux pas! As of yet I haven't found this to be the case, but rules do change, so keep checking in with them.

Room Preparation

Your client has just left and you are getting ready for your next client to show. Hopefully, you have a fifteen minute window where you have sufficient time to clean your room, once the product sales have closed and the niceties are out of the way.

Don't let your idea of housekeeping be 'sweeping' the room with a glance, as housekeeping is something you do that nobody notices, until you *don't* do it!

Remove all sheets and towels used during your last clients visit and dispose of them in the laundry basket. Incidentally all towels and sheets should be washed on a 40°C hot cycle and dried on *high* in the dryer.

All disposable items like spatula's, strips, paper sheeting and gloves should be thrown away immediately so you can begin to wipe down your treatment room ready for the next client to arrive.

Tweezers should be washed with hot soapy water, dried and then immersed in a jar of something that contains all of the ingredients listed below or placed in an autoclave. Every state has different sanitation requirements. Make sure you follow the laws according to where you practice.

Barbicide® is a U.S.A, EPA registered, hospital grade, broad spectrum disinfectant. It is a Germicide, Pseudomonacide, fungicide and virucide. It kills pseudomonas, staph and salmonella. Original Barbicide® also kills HIV – 1 (AIDS virus) Hepatitis B and Hepatitis C on pre-cleaned surfaces and objects previously soiled with blood and bodily fluids. Your tweezers should be immersed for a minimum of ten minutes and it does have an anti-rust formula, so if you leave them in for a bit longer you will not have ruined tweezers.

Wash your hands and begin to prep your room for your next client. Place clean sheets and towels on the bed and set up your table with a clean towel or paper towel ready for your next client. If the paper collar around your waxing pot is very heavily soiled, I would advise you to throw this away and replace with a new one.

If you needed to use the clippers on your client and find that you have tumbleweeds of hair on your tiled floor, starting to resemble a finely crafted rug, sweep up around your area, leaving the floor clean. I specifically mentioned *tiled* floor as carpeting in a waxing room is not advisable due to sanitation and in most states it is against State Board regulations.

If you have a very busy schedule with back to back clients, you may find it easier to layer your bed like a Lasagne! You can drape the bed with a sheet, a towel, then another sheet, a towel and keep adding to the bed draping. This helps to save you on time and a lot of Spa's in high end hotels do this when they have back to back facials or massages.

After each client leaves, remove the sheet and towel that they were laying on and the fresh linens will be on the bed all ready for the next client. This does save time, especially if your linen cupboard isn't in your room but down the corridor.

Some salons that like to save money on the utility bills are happy to just *flip* the sheets and towels over ready for the next client. Please, don't do this. It isn't very sanitary; also sweaty "Eau De Towel" smell isn't appealing to the nose.

Not sure if this story is going to shock you as much as it shocked me when I first heard it......I once had a client who came in to see me for a wax and the first thing that she asked me when she got into the room was "Do you sieve the wax?" I had no clue what she was talking about so I asked her to explain. She told me, that once when leaving a salon after her leg wax; she passed by a side room where the girls appeared to be sieving wax! She explained that they were using sticks to push dripping wax through a sieve back into the wax pot!

They had obviously heated up the *used* hard wax that had been used on previous clients and were straining it through the sieve to re-use the wax and to then throw away the remaining hairs.

I still shudder when I think that this had actually happened and may still be happening. This incident was in America and it was only five years ago that she told me this story. If I ever hear of a salon that does this, I think I would go all loony or "Tabitha" on them and contact State Board of Barbering and Cosmetology.

If your salon that you work at insists that you do this towards helping them cut costs, then I suggest you go find a new place to work. If you are the owner reading this and your salon enforces this rule to save your pocket some money, I suggest you shut the place down and go sit home and wait for Karma to catch up with you!

Fast forward a few months if you will…..

Since, I wrote this chapter a few months ago I actually thought that I was done with talking about sieving wax…. but I have to tell you that this last weekend I taught a back waxing class in Southern California. The student who was attending my class told me that the girl who rents the aesthetician room on a part-time basis in the salon puts the hard wax straight back into the pot after her client has left! Sieving wax through a strainer is one thing, *but actually putting the whole thing back in there is the nastiest thing I have ever heard*! I couldn't believe that after finishing this chapter on this very topic that I was alerted once more about this gross and nasty practice. Of course I was in disbelief, and I had to see this with my own eyes. She took me into the room next door and showed me the wax pot that was not in use and was cold in the tin. But there as *plain as the nose on my face* was hard wax that quite clearly had more pubic hair in it, than I have down there! Time for another hot shower I think!

Curious about what products to use?

I am more than happy to answer *any* questions you might have on what: *Products, new companies, uniforms, educators* or *services* I recommend you try to help you advance within your waxing career.

Product Company's change and new products come on the market that I like to experiment with. So feel free to drop me a line and I can share with you what is new and up and becoming in this industry. Plus, you will be gaining information from somebody who is not affiliated with any product companies and whom is not biased in any way.

After all, don't you want to be better than your competition and stay abreast of new things?

You can contact me through my website listed on the back of this book.

The Art of Sales

"Sales", is not a dirty word! Some technicians cringe when they think of the word, *Sales*. Try and erase that word from your vocabulary. If it makes it easier use the word *consult* if that rings better with you. We all think of used car salesmen with cheesy slicked back hair and a plaid suit when we think of sales, but it doesn't have to be that way.

Whenever you are consulting with a client about what you are doing, what products you are using and why you are using them, in effect you are selling to them simply by educating them. When you inform them that you offer other services in your salon, inform them by making polite conversation that you offer this. Again, this is essentially selling. Listen to what your clients tell you and how they respond.

Don't just presume that because you think you have the best aftercare lotion or offer the best facial in town that they are in a position right now to buy. Advise your clients as to why you think they *need* the product or the service and how it would *benefit* them. Don't push; just consult with them as to why it could potentially be beneficial to them.

The same goes with cross-selling services. If you casually mention, "Hey I have thirty minutes to kill before my next client. If your back hair bothers you, we could wax that for you today to save you another visit." Again, don't just presume that his back hair does bother him as you could insult him. You will get lot's of "Sorry, not right now", *or* "Maybe next time I will try it" *or* "Hmm, let me think about it" Don't take it personally when a client say's no to you. If you are truly authentic and consult from the heart this will soon become evident and trust will soon be built.

I once went into a spa that came highly recommended for a skin consultation as I was just looking for a nice aromatic relaxing facial. We were happily sat chatting about this for a good ten minutes and I was warming up to her and ready to schedule my future relaxing Vitamin C facial appointment. But, then she squinted her eyes at my forehead, twisted her nose as if she disapproved, and suggested I get the wrinkles on my forehead dealt with, by booking in for some Botox also!! She was thinking money and I was thinking, "Rude!!" She didn't listen to a word I said and at the same time, she *presumed* that because my poor wrinkles offended her that they offended me also. I felt insulted so my wrinkly forehead and I left her consultation room (head bowed down in shame) without so much as a future appointment or a recommendation from me!

The point I am trying to make is remember the rule: *"You have two ears and one mouth for a reason!"*

When you are cleaning the client and using the numbing

lotion or talking to her about the sugar scrub, tell her why you are using it or why it would benefit her before or after each appointment and that it would be a great take home product for her to buy so that she has it there ready for her next appointment to use. When you walk her out to reception area, leave the product on the counter, again show her what you are recommending she buys today, and if she has any questions, you are there to answer them. If you don't show her the product that you are suggesting, she could potentially walk right out of your door to the local pharmacy/chemist and buy from them instead, or buy a product that is not appropriate for her skin type.

Send out 'thank you' cards if they are a new client. If you are a female aesthetician and your client is male, keep it professional and not cutesy, the last thing you want is some suspicious crazy, rabbit boiling wife to steam into your location or to accuse him at home of inappropriate behaviour. I once worked with a girl who sent out a thank you card to a first time male client. She wrote on the card "Was so nice meeting you last week, looking forward to the next time". His girlfriend found the card in his car and consequently a fight broke out, he was in the dog house for a week and he never returned to the salon again, but did call us to explain the reason about why he wouldn't be returning! So, keep it very professional and not cutesy. Everything you write should be written as if it will be read by a partner of the client.

Keep a cheat sheet on that client with things that they have told you -- maybe their dog's name, or their children's names, etc. So, when they return, you can look back at your cheat sheet and ask them about their dog, "Ruffus" or how little "Willy" did in his piano recital. People love to be remembered. If you do this often enough, it will soon be lodged into your brain about this persons personal life and you won't need to keep referring back to your cheat sheet...unless of course they are updating you on a vacation that they are about to take. Ask them about it when you see them again. It really makes a difference to that person's experience when you show that you care and that you have listened.

Ask them if they would like to be on your mailing list, so that you can keep them posted about special offers, etc. If they have supplied you with their email address on the consultation form, don't just presume that you can bombard them with your newsletters. Ask them first if they would like to receive them. They may say 'no' in which case just use the email as a confirmation use only. Once your client has agreed to receiving newsletters, make sure that you have an "unsubscribe" option on the bottom of it, so they can at any time decide if it's not for them. I am actually very surprised as to how many companies I receive newsletters from that don't have this unsubscribe option. I find it very annoying.

Mention that she will receive a confirmation call the day before her appointment and possibly a confirmation email also. She may have a preference whether it is phone or email. Listen to what she prefers and use the method that she is asking for.

This is also a fantastic time to say, "It was lovely seeing you today. Thank you so much for coming to see me. It is always appreciated and I will see you in four/six weeks time for your next appointment." She will know why you find it important to see her in this time frame as during the clean up you will have told her why. Shake her hand (as remember shaking hands in business at the end of a service shows that you are grateful for the business), smile nicely, and thank her again. Try and keep at least fifteen minutes between each client, to allow for clean up time, sales, and friendly goodbyes!

As a final motivator, remember it's cheaper and easier to keep your existing clients than to find new ones. Therefore, the more clients that return the more productive and profitable your salon will be.

*If you are not taking care of your
clients, your competitor will.
Bob Hooey*

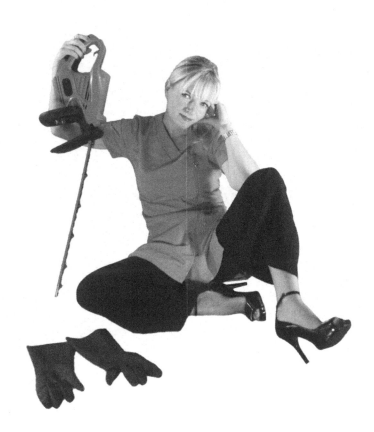

Rewards Programs

Does your salon or spa offer them? Rewards programs are a great way to keep your customers happy and coming back and talking about your place to other people. Some people are so busy focusing on getting new clients that they forget their existing ones. So try some of these reward programs to see what works best for you.

Before she leaves, tell her about the rewards program that you have going on in your salon. For every time she rebooks an appointment and keeps that appointment, she can receive 10% off of her next visit. She can call and change the appointment to another date or time and still get the discount. But, if she cancels with the intention of calling back another day to schedule, then unfortunately she loses the discount. With her knowing this, she is more likely to reschedule there and then on the phone and stick with the appointment.

Give out a handful of your business cards with *her* name written on the back. For every new client that comes to see you with the business card in hand, and her name on the back of it, she then receives a discount for taking the time out and recommending her friends and family to you. Her friends who come in with the business card can also leave with more cards with their name on the back of them also, so that they can also recommend you to their friends and family. It doesn't have to be just for a waxing service; you could offer it for any service that you are licensed or certified to perform in your salon.

If they upgrade their services or try new services, use this as part of the rewards program also. They gain a point for every time they try something new or upgrade. These points can be accumulated over a year. Perhaps they gain five points for referring a friend, or two points for trying a new service etc. At some point once they have collected enough points, which equates to dollars, they could potentially get a service for free! Offering little incentives or reward programs make people feel special. Who doesn't like to be made to feel special?

If your client is a regular who spends a juicy amount of money with you each year, reward them with becoming a silver, gold or platinum member all depending on the dollar amount that they have spent with you each year. With each level that they reach they get discounts or a free hand massage, or free product. The higher the level they reach, the better the reward.

Another option is to give free movie tickets to the client who referred somebody to you. By giving a pair of tickets to your client when she goes to the movies with her friend, her friend will know where the tickets came from, so you will have created another word-of-mouth machine.

If you are cost conscious like we all are these days check with your local cinema to buy a pack of tickets at a discount so you are not paying full face value.

Some salons give away a free pair of knickers for the first time bikini wax client. I think this is a wonderful idea, especially if you offer a range of colors and different sizes to choose from. How wonderful going out that evening on a hot date with your man, all smooth and sexy in the meadows with a brand new pair of knickers on!

There are some companies that offer knickers at wholesale prices with a minimum order of three hundred, where each pair works out to be about $1 a pair. That is a good deal and doesn't chip away too much into your marketing budget.

Most clients don't expect anything, but are very happily surprised when they do receive something. Again you are becoming memorable and irreplaceable *and* they get to go home with leopard print knickers in their handbag! It's a win/win situation for everybody.

As mentioned in the chapter on "How to remove ingrown hairs" you could also send your first time client home with their own personal *knicker sticker* to wear instead of their knickers as a little take home pressie with the hopes that they might *then* buy the pack of seven to use for seven days following their wax.

Please remember my previous comment about informing the client that you are sending them home with a *knicker sticker* simply for the reason that it helps reduce the possibility of getting ingrown hairs and *not* because you are a sloppy waxer that has left big globs of wax in her Garden!

Social Media

I strongly recommend you use social media as one of your marketing tools. By social media, I mean using Twitter, Facebook, YouTube, Blogging, Vlogging, Google+, LinkedIn or Pinterest. These tools are a great way for you to post updates to your fans, followers or contacts about any special offers that your salon may have or any updates about new staff members coming on board. What social media is NOT is a place for you to just sell, sell, and sell. If used correctly, it can greatly increase your profits and credibility. Pinterest as you most probably know is a site where you share pictures with others…this is becoming a fast and furious way to get social and share with others on a different level what interests you.

When using social media as your marketing tool, you are still accountable for keeping your branding alive. You still have a store front at your salon/spa where you engage with clients and people who walk through your door. When people walk through your door at your location, you hopefully show an interest in them while they are visiting. So, sometimes I am left scratching my head as to why people who use social media as their marketing tool ignore their fans or followers.

Engage, engage, and engage. Ask your followers on your

chosen social media site questions and respond to their replies. Maybe you could ask them about their favourite holiday or hobby. It is all about building relationships and showing that you care about them. Ask for their opinions on the blog that you have written. This blog can be attached as part of your newsletter program. Write blogs that are interesting to your industry, mentioning other companies by representing them in a positive manner in your writing. This could be a blog that you have written with your positive thoughts on the wax that you use and why you like it and how it benefits the clients with also including the link to the company's home page in it. This is good marketing for yourself, you are complimenting another company on their product, and positive good energy is spread all around.

With Twitter, you need to tweet consistently to create momentum. Since there is a steady stream of tweets, your tweet can get lost in the active flow of twitters! Twitter is referred to as a cocktail party. Jump in and join conversations. If you find somebody has tweeted something that you find interesting, re-tweet what they have said to *your* followers. When people comment on your tweets or re-tweet something wonderful that you have announced, 'thank' them. Don't ignore them. Remember, if they came into your salon, would you ignore them?

If you were stood alone in a cocktail party trying to make new friends or attract potential clients and all you did was boast about how wonderful you were, or what great offers you had going on in your salon currently, you would notice after a while that the crowd would disperse and you will be left alone munching on the cold cuts. You need to give a piece of *who you are* as this is your branding. People, buy from people they like and trust. How will they know they like you, if all you do is flog your discounted services in their faces every time you are given the opportunity to open your mouth?

So, don't just sell, sell, sell or you may lose your followers and become a bit of a bore. We don't want face-ache nor do we want to appear as a twit-face! Be authentic and post good content that keeps people engaged. When I log onto Twitter and up pops a tweet from a person that I recognize, I smile. I don't always get that feeling if it is a picture of their company logo. I just associate the logo on Twitter with the person trying to sell me something. What makes me feel all fuzzy and wuzzy inside is a person who wants to build relationships with me and cares about me as their potential client. So get your best glamour shot and post it on Twitter…the stream changes so quickly so the more personable you can make it the better.

Twitter has different ways of allowing you to tweet. They have applications like "HootSuite" and many more that allow you to schedule tweets ahead of time. This can save time, but remember to periodically change your scheduled tweets so it stays authentic and doesn't make you appear like a robot or a spam bot.

Facebook is slightly different as your comments; and status stays on the page until you delete it and it doesn't get lost in the flow like it can do on Twitter. Incidentally, don't use your personal/friend page as your business Facebook. Use a 'business' Facebook page and keep it strictly for clients or potential clients. The last thing you need is clients seeing posted pictures of you swinging from a chandelier flashing your knickers off to the cyber world during a night out with the girls in Vegas!

I still think it is great to post good content, ask your fans on your Facebook business page questions, and respond back to their posts. Post updates about special offers that you have, but don't just use this as your *only* way of interacting. If all you do is post special offers, people will start 'hiding' your posts. Occasionally, post a comment about how grateful you are for your fans and how you value them. Update your page daily and be sure to keep it short but sweet. Socialize with them, as that is what social media is all about. It is not 'narcissistic media', if it was, they would call it that. It is not the amount of people you have on Facebook that makes your business effective, it is the amount of 'likes' that you get. This is what gct's you at the forefront of the social media chain!

Check out your local library or book store for books/E-books on social media. Stay ahead of the game and keep up-to-date with newer methods of marketing. This is the future and flyers are pretty much a thing of the past!

Social Media is a great tool for marketing. It is also a great tool for employers to investigate their staff, or new hires. Prior to an interview, make sure your social media sites reflect a professional image of yourself. Some potential employers might check up on you, to see if your profile fits what you have told them in the interview. I do know of some business owners who have done a quick check on potential hires through social media sites. It helps them with the decision making process after an interview. If you don't know what is appropriate, and you wouldn't want your mother to see it, don't post it!

It is also a great tool for employers to use if they have employees, that phone in sick constantly. Make sure your Facebook page from the night before doesn't reflect you having a wild night out. Taking a day off due to a hangover might be a legitimate reason for yourself to be feeling as sick as a dog, whilst barfing down the big white telephone all morning, but your boss won't be on the same page as you! Admittedly, profiles can be blocked preventing the general public from reading it. Make sure yours is blocked if you are a wild cat and especially if you are searching for a new job!

If you feel like being a Twit and want to follow an even bigger Twit, then you can find me on Twitter tweeting from the rooftops @lilbritofwax! Or send me a 'hug' on Facebook and 'like' us https://www.facebook.com/PremierBeautySolutions.

Real Life Stories
from the Experts

I give a certificate to each of my first time Brazilian clients that they all adore written in 'ye old English'. It has a picture of a screaming girl in the corner of the stationary. I then put my arm around them and read it with my best "Queen of England" accent! Jennifer Johnston 'Waxbitch' Michigan USA

This is the certificate I read and give to my clients after they have had a Brazilian. In this the year of our Lord two thousand and twelve, on the _____day of_____in the quaint hamlet of Shaftsburg, under the skillful and steady hands of thy Royal depilation wench, known in this realm as 'Waxbitch', thee fair maiden_____doth bravely and stoically did submit thyself to the most extreme depilatory treatment know to human kind as a 'Brazilian'. Certified by_____ Jennifer Johnston (aka: the Waxbitch)

During the filming of The Secret Life of Brazilian Waxing, we had a couple of male models. Both were a bit nervous of course. One in particular, let's call him "Randy", was very confident that his previous life and training in the Military's, Special Forces had prepared him for the

Brazilian waxing he was about to receive. "I broke my arm jumping out of a plane, If I can handle that, I can handle anything", Randy said confidently. Enter the wax. After the first pull, Randy understood that though the military prepares you to "be all that you can be" it doesn't really prepare you to have the hair ripped out of your bits and pieces. After some whimpering and maybe even a few tears, the job was done. I asked Randy, "So, would you rather have a broken arm, or get another Brazilian?" His response was, "A broken arm". Crickett (The Wax Chick) California.

Over the last 15 years I have learned to adapt to the many different kinds of clients, their levels of pain tolerance and how they cope with being waxed. Many Brazilian first timers deal with waxing like total pros, laying there as I rip the strips, chatting away with excitement about their boyfriend coming back from an 8 month deployment in Afghanistan. Some swear like sailors with each loving pull but when it's all over say, 'it really wasn't that bad, when should I come back for my next appointment'?

Then we have the wax virgins who not only think they are about to be slaughtered but the panic attacks and freak outs begin even as I touch them lightly to prep the skin. These are the clients who I hold hands with when they need a moment to breathe in and out like they are doing Lamaze and assure them its ok they are nervous and it's all going to be ok. This is when my patience and role playing kick in and I become the compassionate caring nurse, supportive best friend and cheerleader. Before I pull a strip that may be one of the more 'ouchie' ones I tell them to go their happy place and often suggest they are running in a field with puppies and kittens.

Some clients close their eyes tight and immediately head for the pasture of furry love and others will say' but I don't like kittens', so I'll say 'ok there are only puppies in your happy place, the puppies chased all those horrible little kitties away'. I can also get a good laugh from them when they are in their most vulnerable position on their hands and knee's or what I like to call 'downward dog'. It's at this special and intimate moment I tell them to just 'pretend' I'm not here'. So as I begin to wipe warm wax between their cheeks they can giggle as to what a silly thing I just suggested! Jennifer Johnston 'Waxbitch' Michigan USA

This isn't a waxing story but it does involve a client who complained about me to my manager/owner of the salon that I worked for a few years ago. I am also a nail technician as well as an aesthetician and one day this guy sits down in my chair ready for his pedicure. I proceed to start chatting with him by asking him how his day was going until he firmly says "I am not here to talk, why do you girls always insist on talking to me and presuming that is what I want?" I was floored, as I was only trying to make him feel comfortable five minutes into his appointment as the foot spa was heating up. For the rest of the service, I did as he requested and didn't start conversation again. He waited after his appointment for twenty minutes until the owner came back from lunch, so that he could complain about how rude I was, and how unwelcome I made him feel etc.... NOW that is one nut job if you ask me!! Sometimes you just cannot win with some people! Claire Barnes. Author.

We once had a client who came in for a wax (I was the receptionist) and she insisted that her boyfriend be there with her in the room during the wax. The room was so small with barely enough room for the Esthetician doing the service that day, but she insisted he stayed. It took our Esthetician longer than it should have done with him pressed against the trash can, trying not to get in the way, made her unfortunately lose her cool. She refused to carry on with the service until he left the room as it was making her job harder. Both of them decided this wasn't a professional place to get a service so abruptly they got up and left! She had half of her bikini waxed, didn't offer to pay for time wasted and fled the salon! We felt our Esthetician was justified in her actions and made that our new policy in our salon. Jeanette Beasingdale. U.K

A bikini wax that should have just taken me fifteen minutes to do, actually took me over thirty minutes. My client kept hopping out of the room every few minutes to visit the ladies room. Apparently after her third visit to the ladies room she informs me her next appointment for the day was to go to the Doctor's as she suspected she had a bladder infection! I think a visit to the Doctor's office and a shot of Cranberry juice should have happened before a waxing appointment! Veni Larkin. Chicago. U.S.A (The Green Spa)

Have you ever tried to wax a client's eyebrows when they don't shut their eyes? Her beady eyes were constantly staring right up at me the whole time. Was kinda freaky if you ask me. I did ask her to close her eyes to avoid any wax accidentally blobbing into her eyeballs, but she seemed so tense watching my every move. I feel like it was the worst eyebrow wax I have ever done. I never saw Miss Beady eye again...that was strange in a psychotic way! Carla Rees. Orange County. Ca

I was once asked out on a date by a client at beauty school when I was waxing his back. He told me he was sexually aroused and my touch turned him on. "Get out you little s**t" was what I wanted to say. I politely told him his service was over and he needed to get dressed and leave. Ugh! Danielle Westbrook. Austin. Texas. (Student)

At beauty school we were selected to do services on clients on a number basis. When the teacher shouted your number you knew it was your turn to take the next client without question. This client had come in for a bikini wax and I had only observed before and had never actually waxed one. I panicked, totally freaking out and wanting to cry. I took the client back to my station area asking her if it was her first time. It turned out she was an Esthetician and was actually 'head hunting' students with the hopes of hiring students once graduated and licensed to work in her new spa that was opening a few months later. I confessed to her that she was my first bikini wax and I didn't know what I was doing! She guided me through the whole thing and it was like having my own private lesson. I never did get hired at her new place, but it was the best learning experience I had and I am forever grateful! Danielle Westbrook. Austin. Texas (Student)

I was new to the spa and new to the industry. We decided to place an ad looking for 'non-paying' clients so that I could get some practice. One guy responded by email with "Tall, very handsome and extremely athletic" will be interested in getting a waxing service. I did think it slightly 'odd' that he would actually write that about himself as I wasn't putting an ad out there for dating, but for waxing. He showed up the following week for his appointment. He was "Short and ugly with nothing athletic about him at all!" I waxed him with a smile on my face wondering how he could get his description so wrong! Dee Dee. San Diego. Ca

I once had a client who came into the salon that spoke very little English. He informed me that he was Russian and that he had done some research on-line about the man waxing. Throughout the service, I kept telling her that he needed to hold herself so I could wax easier around her. He kept letting go and proudly showing me his man parts. I started to get slightly angry and was just about ready to tell her to get dressed and leave my room, which in this profession we are within our rights to end a service at any time if we feel uncomfortable. I firmly told her that he needed to do this to make it easier on both of us but he didn't. So, I got out my tweezers and started to tweeze the hairs from his testes. Ouch! He soon lost his manhood and soon didn't seem to find it pleasurable anymore. I ended his service; he lay there all confused when I told her it was over. His comment was, "Huh is that it?" "Don't I get anything else?" in his stupid broken English. Not sure what website he had been looking at but he certainly wasn't getting it in my salon!! By the way, I never got a tip either...tight ass!! -- Lesley MacArthur, USA

I came into work one morning (slightly hung-over from the night before from the staff Xmas party!). The receptionist said "Oh, you have a client on his way that is requiring a waxing from you." "What sort of waxing does he want?" I asked. "He was very vague on the phone and said he would explain it to you when he arrived." Strange! So I waited for my client who showed up larger than life all jolly and ready to go. I took her into my room and asked her what sort of wax did he want? "I really just want the bottom part doing" He tells me. "Ok, Sir, undress from the waist down and I will be back in the room shortly" I tell her. I come back in to find this rather large, heavy set gentleman on all fours on my bed with his bum cheeks spread apart! All he wanted was an anus wax! It was 8am, I was hung-over, I had just eaten a greasy breakfast and I wanted to die! -- Sally Jensen, UK

A really pretty female came in for a bikini wax. She was a college, student and very chatty. I waxed around the sides of her bikini area...piece of cake. As I started to wax around the sides of her labia, I came across something that I had never seen before. I wasn't too sure what it was, but it resembled a cluster of blisters. It looked pretty sore, so I asked her about it. "Don't worry about it, I am pretty resilient to pain...it's a Herpes outbreak, that I get once a year!" WTH? Obviously, I told her I shouldn't/couldn't wax around that area as the likelihood of it spreading is very high. Thank goodness for latex gloves (that I was wearing) and get this!!!! I had to throw the whole pot of wax away as this was five or six years ago when double dipping was never known to be an issue!!! Expensive service for me that was!!!! -- Sian Cooke, UK

A marine just home from his deployment was coming in for a back wax before he visited his girlfriend that he hadn't seen for nine months. He was telling me during *the prepping process that he was in Afghanistan and that things were brutal, but he enjoys it and just misses his family. As I start to wax, he yelps out and nearly flies off the bed! He hated every minute of it and told me it was the most painful thing he had ever experienced! Military back packs, military boots, trudging through the hot sweltering heat and this was more painful!! Hmmmm! -- Denise, USA*

I was waxing a guy who flew his legs around the bed every time I tried to wax them which was pretty disturbing.... Or, maybe it was the fact that his lip gloss was shinier than mine...not sure! – Kimberly, Vancouver, Canada

In regards to how 'vulnerable' men feel when getting waxed, here's a great story!!! In October I got a call from Afghanistan. It was a U. S. Marine telling me he'd been over there for almost a year in the mountains and he was 'dirty, hairy and wanted a full body wax' when he got back in December. I asked him how the heck he got my number and he said, 'Your website'. The internet truly connects the world! Anyways, when he finally came in for his appointment, he told me he had only ever waxed himself but had never attempted a Brazilian for obvious reasons. As he was on his hands and knees with his bum in the air he was kind of mumbling and then he said quietly, 'I don't think I have ever been more vulnerable in my entire life, um, uh, I think this may just be worse than 9 months in Afghanistan.'

At the end of it all, he was thrilled with the results and headed out for a 'hot date'. I now have an amazing testimonial but one new clients would not appreciate....'Waxbitch' worse than 9 months in Afghanistan'. I may have a future in terrorist interrogations!!! Jennifer Johnston 'Waxbitch' Michigan USA

Questionnaire filled out...all complete. Check all boxes. No Retin-A or Acutane. Perfect. Rip! Talk about lifting the skin!! Practically half her eye-lid was removed! She did confess that she took Retin-A, but was embarrassed to admit to it! She was pissed with ME!!! I told her that the paperwork told her the reasons why the questions were being asked. – Anonymous

A few years back I had a very jumpy male client in for his first ever Brazilian wax. Despite a few nervous twitches on the front, all went well until I flipped him over onto his knees and elbows so that I could remove the hair from his backside. With my customer on all fours and his bottom up in the air, I duly slapped wax all over his bum cheeks and laid my first paper strip, ready for the off. Bracing the skin tightly, I proceeded to pull the strip off as per normal... whereupon my client yelped like a wounded animal and leapt forward on the treatment couch. With visions of him diving headfirst off the end of the bed and my career in tatters, I did what any self-respecting therapist in a blind panic would do: I rugby tackled him around the thighs. There was a moment of awkward silence where it slowly dawned on both of us that my cheek was now firmly stuck to his cheek, so to speak, before (fortunately) he started laughing. On the plus side, at least I didn't have a beard, and he's still a customer to this day... although I've since learned to warn clients before tugging the wax off!! Andy Rouillard. Axiom Bodyworks. U.K

I do full male Brazilians (that's the whole kit-and-kaboodle from the pubic bone to the tailbone and every wobbly bit in between) I had a man call and ask if getting a Brazilian was like a massage or like going to the Doctor. I wish I had responded with, 'Well that depends If you think having your hair ripped from your scrotum and bum is a massage.' but I was a good girl/professional and just bluntly said, 'going to the Doctor' and he thanked me and I never heard from him again!!!! LOL Jennifer Johnston 'Waxbitch' Michigan USA

I have never had any awkward issues with my male Brazilian clients because they come to me knowing it's a professional waxing service and nothing else. (My website states this also) Due to the fact I have a home salon, male clients must be accompanied by a female or I take males coming alone when my husband is in the house (my hubby does not make it obvious he's home because I'm not trying to intimidate my male clients either, just playing it safe) Many will come with their girlfriends or wives (although there for moral support, it usually ends up with them trying not to laugh as their 'boo' is on his hands and knees.)

I always make the male client feel like this is no big thing and I do this all day long. They see that I am friendly but confident and in control by giving them directions throughout....'pull your penis over to the right, left, toward the belly button, pull your scrotum up, over...I start all my male clients on their knees and wax their bum first because I feel it lets them know who is in charge right from the beginning. Jennifer Johnston 'Waxbitch' Michigan USA

I had a brand new client who was leaving the next day for vacation and had NEVER had a bikini or Brazilian wax before. She came in nervous and sweaty. At the time, I was using an awful green wax (forgot the name of it). Needless to say, it clumped up in her hair and matted everything together, so I put hard wax on top of the clumped up green wax mess and it turned to a ball of glue. Scissors came out next, clumps of hair, bleeding, sweat and body odour.... two hours later. – Stephanie G Laynes, USA*

A wife made an appointment for her husband's back to be waxed and he had never had a wax before. I suggested that the hair be about no more than an inch long and to try and cut it prior to the appt. This big, burly man walked into the room and was little uneasy but was ready to have the wax service. After the first rip, sweat starting rolling down is back and forehead. He asked me for a towel to hold onto cause he gets sweaty when he is nervous, so I handed him a towel and he began to bite on it and shake. After the second rip, he kept the towel in his mouth and grabbed the underside of the massage bed with both arms. After the third rip, he begged me to go to his wife to get some drugs. Needless to say, his wife was waiting with the pills in hand mumbling about him being a FIREFIGHTER. – Stephanie G Laynes, USA*

During beauty school, my friend Tina and I decided to partner up in the eyebrow wax class. She was pretty proficient in make up application so I thought I would let her go first. One eyebrow was completed as she stood back, hands on hips proudly examining her work!! I was very happy and hummed to myself as she started on the second one. I was going to like my new designer brows.

She proceeded to wax, then stopped and gasped! There was a long period of silence. "Ms. Jay", she yelled across the room, "Come quickly." I sat upright..."What? What?" I asked. Ms. Jay comes over and calmly informs us that it's nothing an eyebrow pencil cannot correct. Tina had waxed my brow with a wax strip that had wax on it from the previous brow. As she placed it over my brow the wax removed a huge chunk right out of the centre of my brow!!! I was due to go on holiday to Greece for a few weeks a week later and I travelled very closely with my new eyebrow pencil!!! -- Claire Barnes. Author

We got a phone call once at the salon from a very irate mother who complained bitterly that her daughter, who was only 16, had come in to see us for a Brazilian bikini wax. My manager was off sick this day so being the head aesthetician I took the call. She was devastated that we would wax a girl that young (hey lady, it's your daughter going to the prom with other thoughts on her mind... saucy minx). She said she had gone to school that day very uncomfortable and with a very bad rash spreading around her voojie. I asked her what her daughter was wearing for school that day and she told me that she was wearing jeans. I told the angry mother on the phone very calmly that wearing jeans would irritate her even more and could she bring her in after school, so I could take a look at her. She agreed, but they never showed up that day or the next. I called the lady with a concerned follow-up call and she humbly apologized and told me on her way to the salon that her daughter told her she had called the wrong salon! I thought when I checked the books that there was no person with that name on there, but with divorced parent's, who knows these days, who, is called what. I do wish the angry lady would have taken it upon herself to call us back and apologize for accusing us of something we had never done!! -- Jennifer Boneo, USA

I had on my books an hour-and-a half massage, (it happens once a year, the most people want around here is an hour) so I was so extremely excited, that I completely forgot, that I had just one 'little' bikini wax to do before that appointment.

I set up, lit the candles, the client came, filled out a form, then I took her to the room, showed her around and told her basically, just leave your panties on, and lay face down under the blanket.....

I waited a little and entered the room; she is in the bed facing down undressed. She looks up at me and said "This is just a regular bikini right?

I looked at her "Well, had you not said anything, you would have got an hour and a half massage!!" She has been coming to me for years for bikini waxing; she even took her shirt off!!

She said "Well, I know you know what you are doing; I thought maybe there is a new way of doing it!"

We have been laughing about it ever since!

Just shows how much power you gain by earning your client's trust! *Eva Walker. Soul Escape, Esthetics Day Spa. BC. Canada*

Real Life Stories
from Clients

I made the trek to a well-known wax studio -- a place that was heavily frequented by celebrities. The owner was a bit of her celebrity herself since she worked with so many of them. Once she started on my wax, we were making small talk and she asked me how I came to find her. I told her that I heard about her on the news from a local weather girl. That sent her into a tailspin and she started telling me why this weather girl doesn't come to her anymore. The story went on for some time and she actually stopped waxing me and sat on the table next to me. If that wasn't bad enough, she took the muslin cloth that she had just ripped off of me and laid it on her thigh while she finished the story. Now I know it was my hair on the muslin but I really didn't want to look at it. She simmered down and finished. She had my flip to do the back side and when she was all done gave me a little slap on the booty. Totally creepy and totally unprofessional and I never returned. – Cassie Piasecki, USA

I had a God-forsaken eyebrow wax with a technician who constantly kept popping gum in her mouth as she leant over me trying to wax my brows. Her gum chewing was obviously trying to mask the smell of nicotine...totally gross and not at all professional. No return for me! -- P. Chadwick, USA

There's nothing worse than going to a salon, whether it's for hair, waxing or facials and the person working on you compares themselves to their competition down the street! Not interested...but the one thing I will do is try out your competition as they have to be waaay more professional than you!! -- Mary Venderbilt, USA

I was having a good day until I went for my monthly lip wax. The usual place I went to was closed for a few weeks following some severe water pipe leakage...so I tried some random place. As she starts to wax my lip, she steps back with her face and asks me if I had ever considered Botox for the lines around my mouth as I needed it! Hmm!!! -- Sarah Mancini, USA

I went on my fantastic honeymoon with three hickies around my bikini area! They were not from a night of sex but a drastic bikini wax a few days before! It was a case of ..... Apply the wax, stand back, and just pull it without holding me. I cried when I got home, but being the big baby that I am, I never said anything in the salon. Chicken I know! ☹ -- Toni Lavacot, Orange County, California

There's nothing worse than having a technician who huffs and puffs due to their frustrations at working on my bikini hair! OK, OK, I know its super coarse...some have told me I am very difficult! I have now found a great gal who does an amazing job and seems to enjoy the challenge I bring to her every month! -- Ruby, USA

I had a gal get wax stuck in my belly button once from my chest and stomach wax. When she got the metal plucking things out to remove it, I decided going home and taking

a shower would be safer. My wife would help me remove the big blob I am sure. -- James Moore, USA

I went in for a back wax and the lady used a roller type of device. It looked like a big glue stick but had wax drip out the end. Well, she put the wax on, but it wouldn't come off. She said the wax was probably a bit too cold, so kept going over it and over it to remove it. In the end she had to pick most of it off! I felt bad for her as she was new out of school and seemed a bit upset. When I voiced my concerns nicely to the receptionist who also happened to be the manager, then that was a different story. Apparently, it was my fault as I must have had dry skin!! Ok, lady....I didn't go back to your dumb place again. -- Frank Parish, Vancouver, Canada

I had dark blue hard wax stuck up my nostril once! Having a stranger pick your nose was an experience I won't forget! It came out eventually with most of my brain I think! -- Mike G, USA

I went to Las Vegas with the boys for a long weekend last year. So I decided I would have more chance of finding the chicks if I had my vest removed! I broke out like a teenager!! I had more pimples than I have ever had in my life!! Pretty common I heard with some waxes. I have been back a few times since as I heard your skin needs to get used to it. It did get a bit better, but not worth it. Not for me. The chicks will have to like me hairy! -- Anonymous

I will tell you what I don't like when I see somebody in a salon. Drama! All some of them do is yack, yack, yack. When my eyes are closed, I am probably meditating

through the leg wax, as I admit, I find it painful! But, when you continue to yack for an hour solid about your life and your boyfriend, it makes it more painful!! Ok, I will shut up now. Thanks for allowing me to write my vent! -- Marie W., London, U.K.

I was once told that I had a really nice vagina! Nice! I wasn't sure what to make of that comment, but I will keep the compliment, thank you very much! -- Anonymous

I wasn't too sure why when I sometimes got a leg wax did I come out feeling stubbly. I never knew why until an esty told me it was because the paper wasn't removed correctly and I might has well have stayed home and shaved as the hair roots were still in there. Please remember girlies, I paid for a leg wax, not a shave. -- Irritated in Orange County, USA

I had a bikini wax in beauty school once. I say once, because I never did it again!! They had to get the scissors out to remove the wax that was all stuck to my pubic hair. The wax felt cold and I always thought it was hot wax that is used. Not sure what went wrong and I feel bad as they are all students...but the teacher was on the missing list. I was sore for about a week after that. Ugh. -- Phillipa Adkins, Washington, USA

I hate, hate having my feet waxed. Its part of the full leg wax...but the darn stuff never comes off the tops of my feet!! -- Anonymous

I haven't had any really, really bad experiences. For the most part, I love visiting the salon for a wax. I am much

happier now also that most places don't double dip. I never gave it much thought before until the girl who waxes me proudly told me it was their policy. -- Sarah Green, UK

Was looking forward to a leg wax with a new girl that the salon advised I try. The whole time she waxed me, she kept complaining about how her boss was a b***h, how she never got adequate lunch breaks. I was stressed, just listening to her! Please, don't tell me your salon politics, I have enough of my own to deal with in my own office!! -- Mary Beddington. Orange County, California

It took me a while to find somebody who did an efficient bikini wax, and once when visiting L.A I came across a great place owned by a British woman. They did a great job....wish they had a place in Colorado where I live! -- Tina Alcala, Denver.

I was in Tenerife on holiday and decided to go to the local chemist and buy a pot of cold wax. It was a funky green colour and was applied cold. Trying to get the stuff off was a nightmare and I was left with bruises and sore patches of skin. Not to forget a sunburn as I had to walk back to the chemist with green funk still attached to my legs, to see if they had a product that I could use to remove it. All of a sudden their English wasn't too good and they acted dumb! I fumbled my way back to the hotel where I spent the next 3 hours using everything from baby oil to hot showers trying to release the stuff from my legs. The first wax I ever had was not done by a professional but by me! I eventually got it all off, minus a few sheets of skin and still hairy legs!! My next wax will certainly be done by a professional. Mary V Pinnock. Leicester. U.K

Glossary of British Terms

- Aunt Flow – Menstrual Cycle
- Big White Telephone – Toilet
- Bob's your Uncle – As easy as that
- Bit's and Bob's – Thing/Things
- Brilliant – Awesome
- Buggers – Nuisance things
- Bum – Butt
- Cheeky – Sassy
- Choccies - Chocolates
- Crabby – Bitchy
- Dingle Berries – Poop
- Dithering – Awkwardly fussing around things
- Ferret – Rummage around
- Freebie - Free
- Handbag – Purse
- Jiffy – In a minute
- Knickers – Underwear
- Lady Garden – Vagina
- Loo – Bathroom/Restroom
- Love Bite – Hickey
- Nappy - Diaper
- Pressie - Gift
- Tacky – Sticky
- Tackle –His junk down there
- Tid-Bits – Pieces of

- Tooting Gas - Farting
- Trousers - Pants
- Verbal Diarrhoea – Overflow of mindless chatter
- Wotsits – Your you-know-what
- Waffling – see Verbal Diarrhoea